The Student Nurse Guide to Decision Making in Practice

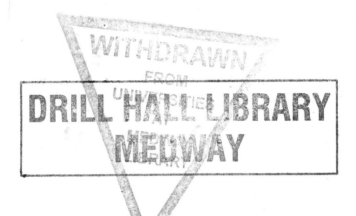

The Student Nurse Guide to Decision Making in Practice

Edited by
Liz Aston, Jill Wakefield and Rachel McGown

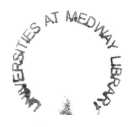

Open University Press

Open University Press
McGraw-Hill Education
McGraw-Hill House
Shoppenhangers Road
Maidenhead
Berkshire
England
SL6 2QL

email: enquiries@openup.co.uk
world wide web: www.openup.co.uk

and Two Penn Plaza, New York, NY 10121—2289, USA

First published 2010

Copyright © Liz Aston, Jill Wakefield and Rachel McGown 2010

A catalogue record of this book is available from the British Library

ISBN-13: 978-0-33-5236640
ISBN-10: 0-33-523664-2

Typeset by Kerrypress, Luton, Bedfordshire
Printed and bound in the UK by Bell and Bain Ltd., Glasgow

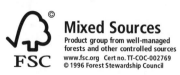

Mixed Sources
Product group from well-managed
forests and other controlled sources
www.fsc.org   Cert no. TT-COC-002769
© 1996 Forest Stewardship Council
FSC

The McGraw·Hill Companies

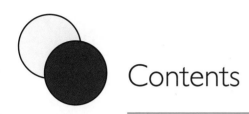

Contents

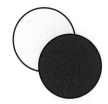

Figures

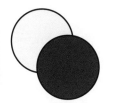

Tables

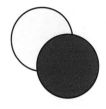

Praise for this book

I found this book extremely easy to read and use ... The book covers all pre-registration nursing branches and can be used throughout the degree course and into registered nursing. I will use this book throughout the remainder of my Nursing Degree and beyond, and would recommend it to my peers.

Conor Hamilton, Student Nurse, Queens University Belfast, UK

This book is extremely enjoyable to read. The material covered is easy to follow as well as being informative, while highlighting key areas that are important to a student nurse. The clear diagrams and style of writing are superb. The practical and real life exercises take this book to the next level and make a heavy subject enjoyable and educational. The fact the book is directed to all areas of nursing make this a must have guide for all student nurses.

Lisa Perraton, Student Nurse, University of Chester, UK

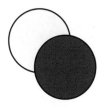

About the Editors

Liz Aston

Liz Aston started nurse training in 1972 and qualified in 1975 and has worked in a variety of acute care as well as rehabilitation settings. She entered education as a clinical teacher in the 1980s and has always maintained an active interest in practice learning issues. She is currently Associate Professor and Lead for Practice Learning in the Division of Nursing at the University of Nottingham.

Jill Wakefield

Jill Wakefield qualified as an adult nurse in 1979 and worked for a number of years in an adult intensive care setting. Having developed an interest in helping others to learn, she became a clinical teacher at the Nottingham School of Nursing in January 1986 and later a tutor at 1991 and has continued in this role to the present. Her areas of interest centre on nursing management issues (especially those related to senior students). Other areas of interest reflect clinical links with cardiac and diabetic care.

Rachel McGown

Rachel McGown has worked in acute medicine, elderly care settings and as a nurse practitioner. She has also had experience as a practitioner health lecturer at the University of Nottingham. She is currently working in health care of the older person as a deputy ward manager.

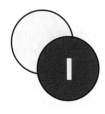

Making the transition to student nurse

Introduction

From a very early age, we all make decisions of one kind or another. A child will perhaps decide that he or she is not going to eat the green vegetables put before them at dinner time. When asked why, the reply may be 'because I don't like them!' This is a decision without much reasoning. Now consider a young adult – they may well decide that they will eat their green vegetables that are served to them at dinner time. This is a different decision about a similar situation but if you ask the young adult why they are going to eat their green vegetables, their response might well be ' … because they are good for me!' What has happened in the intervening period of time from child to young adulthood?

The young adult will have learned the art of reasoning, through knowledge acquisition, experiences, the influence of family and social circles, school, college, work, and so on. These influences are very important in guiding people to make decisions and obviously the quality of this input will lead to varying degrees of success in decision making.

Exercise 1.1

You have made a decision that you want to take a holiday in France. What will you need to do to ensure that your trip is successful?

On thinking about this, you will find that this is a complex decision, particularly if you have never been abroad before. Do you have a valid passport? If not, this can take some time to organize. Where in France do you want to go? What do you know about France? Can you speak any French? How are you going to get there? Are you going to stay in a hotel or a self-catering apartment? Can the Internet help? The list is probably endless but the point being made here is that successful decision making requires sophisticated reasoning in order to avoid a disaster!

Responsibility and accountability

As adults, we are all expected to be responsible (i.e. not reckless). We know that we should not drink over the permitted level of alcohol if we are going to drive a car but why do some people continue to do this? This is an example of recklessness. All adults are constantly made aware of the dangers of drinking and driving and the effects of alcohol on the body. If you are stopped by the police and breathalyzed and you are over the limit, you can expect to be dealt with by the legal process – you are both responsible and accountable to the law of the land (and indeed the fellow public!) However, as a health professional, your responsibility and accountability have a much wider scope. Figure 1.1 illustrates this.

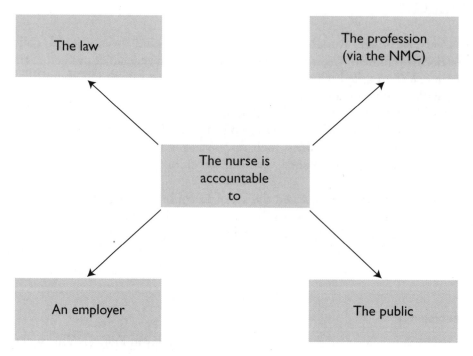

Figure 1.1 Accountability as a nurse

The public

We have accountability to ensure that the public when they present themselves in a health care setting is assured of a competent, caring, trustworthy and professional approach from a qualified nurse. As a student you need to be aware that you will be working towards this. The public see a nurse in a uniform and do not take account of the fact that you are a student. This means that you must demonstrate a caring and professional approach. Any limitations that you consider may affect your competence in a situation must be referred back to the qualified nurse for advice.

Our employer

We have accountability to ensure that as nurses, we work within the policies, guidelines and procedures specified by our employers. In addition, we need to work co-operatively with all members of the health care team who are employed within our work settings. As a student, although not an employee, you also need to be aware of those policies, procedures and guidelines particularly as students work across different areas.

The professional body – Nursing and Midwifery Council (NMC)

We are accountable to our professional body and to follow the standards set out in the *The Code* (NMC, 2008). As a student you need to follow these standards as advised in *Guidance on Professional Conduct for Nursing and Midwifery Students* (NMC, 2009).

The law

We are ultimately accountable to the law of the country in which we work; in addition, if that country is part of the European Union (EU), we are also accountable to the European courts. This also applies to students.

The NMC (2008: 1) specifies that: '… as a professional you are personally account-able for actions and omissions in your practice and must always be able to justify your decisions': As a student, you need to work towards this, hence the requirements to understand the reasons for decisions made.

It is clear from this outline that any decisions that you make as a nurse are going to have repercussions in a number of areas. These might include:

- **Public:** going home in your uniform and witnessing a collapse. You did not intervene due to your not feeling competent to deal with this situation. It is perceived by the public as being uncaring and unprofessional, and a witness may well report you for this.
- **Employer:** when transferring a patient from one surface to another, the policy specifically states that a sliding sheet must be used to ensure a smooth and safe transfer. You fail to use the sliding sheet because it involves some extra effort in

terms of finding the sliding sheet. This is in direct contravention of an agreed and evidenced policy and could place a patient at risk of harm.

- **Professional body:** you have been out to a celebration party and have consumed a good deal of alcohol. You returned to your home in the early hours of the morning but only manage to get three hours sleep before you have to get up to go to an early shift in your current clinical placement. You are not going to feel fit enough for what could be a very demanding shift and your thinking processes are likely to be impaired. This clearly goes against the NMC Code requirements (NMC, 2008).
- **Law:** not recording care given and, as a student, not getting it countersigned by a registered nurse. Should this record be scrutinized, it will be deemed that if the care was not recorded, it was not given. It would be impossible to prove subsequently that indeed this care was given.

We have written this book to help enable you to be effective in your decision making during your nursing career and to understand the reasoning behind it.

How nurses are expected to make decisions about a client's care

In making care decisions, the nurse has to balance a number of elements. First and foremost is acting in the client's best interests. This is straightforward when a client is able to voice their views on their care, but there are many instances where this may not be possible. Other influences will impinge on the nurse's decisions.

Family and relatives

For example, the patient's family and relatives: the nurse often has to balance the wishes of the patient's family and relatives and the patient themselves when making a care decision. Sometimes, this can lead to conflict; an example of this is where a patient wishes to return to their own home but the family and relatives know that the patient will not be able to cope there and they are unable to provide any additional support. In such a case, the nurse would have to try and make arrangements to suit all parties but often this is not possible.

Where other carers are involved, whether they be formal or informal, it is often the case that they need to be consulted when making a care decision. For instance, a patient with learning disabilities may be admitted to an acute ward in a hospital. It is vital to involve that patient's carer in decisions, particularly if invasive treatment is contemplated. There could be problems with communication and consent that only the patient's regular carer may be able to overcome.

Resources

Resources are increasingly an issue for a nurse when clinical decision making is required. An example of this might occur when patients need to be moved and equipment is required to enable this (i.e. a hoist). There is a variety of hoisting equipment on the market and one of the problems is finding a hoist that will cope with different moving situations. Such a hoist is likely to be expensive and with financial restrictions, this situation can be very difficult in making a satisfactory decision. It may well be that a trust keeps a stock of equipment to be loaned out for difficult situations, but the supply is likely to be restricted and hoists such as this may be required simultaneously in different locations.

Satisfying all parties

It is sometimes difficult for the nurse to come to a decision that will satisfy all parties – the important element in all of this is that the nurse is able to justify the decision. As a student, you will be guided by your mentors with regard to this until you reach the final stages of your pre-registration course. A good strategy to employ in the early stages of the course is to discuss with your mentor how you can justify a decision that you have jointly made. As you proceed through your course, you will be expected to increasingly demonstrate your knowledge when making decisions; you will also be expected to utilize up-to-date evidence to support your decisions and also to work within the policies and procedures of your clinical areas.

There is no doubt that nursing has developed its professional role in recent times. In addition, the accompanying advancements in science and technology in health care have made the remit of the nurse far more complex. Constant reforms and political involvement in the National Health Service (NHS) have added to this. Nurses have a great deal to contend with in the way of meeting targets, patient outcomes, and many nurses now take on roles formerly held by medical staff, and the reduction in junior doctors' working hours is but one example of how this has affected the nursing workload and accompanying responsibility and accountability. The question should be posed as to how this affects nurses' decision making about a client's care. The developments described above greatly influence decision making. Think about the influences on a common nursing decision.

Exercise 1.2

A nurse decides to place a patient on a pressure-relieving airflow mattress to prevent the development of pressure sores:

  What might have led the nurse to make this decision?

  What are the implications of this action?

  What other decisions need to be made to help prevent the development of a pressure sore?

There will be a number of factors that will have influenced the nurse to make the above decision. These are likely to be:

- An assessment tool to identify the risk of a patient developing a pressure sore should have been used.
- The nurse must be able to use that tool correctly. There is a need to develop effective clinical judgement in order to do this. Flow diagrams produced in conjunction with pressure sore assessment tools can help nurses in this respect.
- The use of pressure-relieving equipment often implies expense; for instance, the hiring of such equipment, running costs and maintenance. There is a need to fully justify the use of such equipment. Again, flow charts can assist nurses to select the most effective and economic equipment and these are now based on best evidence.
- Good nutrition to promote tissue health and repair is also necessary; without this, other measures will not be effective.
- Changing of position and exercises (passive or active) to keep the circulation of blood effective.
- Thought needs to be given to the patient who, while nursed on an airflow mattress in bed, is transferred to a chair for a time. Other equipment is needed to address the issue of pressure relief while the patient is seated in the chair. Failure to consider this will negate the beneficial effects of the airflow mattress.

In addition, the nurse's knowledge and use of evidence should have played a part in this decision. Later chapters will address the issues around knowledge and evidence:

- Chapter 3: Using evidence to support decision making (i.e. selecting varied and effective evidence)
- Chapter 4: Getting the most out of your mentor (i.e. learning from role models)
- Chapter 7: Increasing complexity in decision making (i.e. expanding knowledge).

All these chapters will guide your development in making decisions.

It is evident therefore that the qualified nurse in making decisions about a client's care is expected to utilize valid evidence to support those decisions; to utilize resources cost-effectively; to ensure that such resources are used correctly for a patient; and indeed that other care staff do the same. The qualified nurse can expect to be challenged at any point about his or her decisions for patient care and will be held to account for them in a number of areas. All this implies that the qualified nurses must keep themselves up to date in their area of practice and always be prepared to extend and deepen their knowledge and experience in order to be effective decision-makers. This is why it is necessary for you, as a student, to learn the skills of decision making.

An introduction to decision making theory

For some time there has been evidence in the nursing literature concerning models and discourses relating to decision making theory. In order to help you appreciate and understand these aspects, the principal theories of decision making are now going to be introduced.

The information-processing model

The underpinning element of this model concerns how information is stored and retrieved. In our life, we acquire information from a variety of sources; most information is stored in the long-term memory due to its larger capacity. The sources of information come from learning in education as well as other settings, as a result of life experiences, socialization and employment. Initially, such information will be stored in the short-term memory but eventually it will find its way into the long-term memory. In fact, you will probably learn about this in the behavioural sciences component of your nursing course. Application of this model in nursing may be seen when a nurse assesses a patient for the first time – information is gained and immediately placed in the short-term memory. This then 'triggers' certain cues that cause information retrieval from the long-term memory.

Chest pain = MI

The intuition model

Intuition may be defined as 'the power of the mind by which it immediately perceives the truth of things without reasoning or analysis'. The intuition model of decision making is more readily connected with the work of expert nurses and this may be seen where a nurse can quickly make a decision concerning patient care having had a great deal of previous experience in a certain type of care. The term 'gut feeling' has been applied (Muir, 2004). For instance, an experienced nurse working in a respiratory care setting may observe a patient experiencing a severe asthma attack. A wheeze is present and should this disappear, the experienced nurse will know instinctively that this can signify a serious deterioration in the patient's state and will be prompted to make further checks on the patient that can result in the decision to call the emergency team. Previous situations will have caused this experienced nurse to recognize that there may be a problem immediately; hence the use of the term 'intuition'.

The cognitive continuum theory

Intuition and information processing may be regarded as two ends of a spectrum as a means of decision making. In reality, most nurses utilize a mixture of the two elements in their decision making. A model has been proposed to take account of this situation: the cognitive continuum theory. Cader et al. (2005) have explained that this theory involves six broad modes of decision making and that the continuum varies from intuition to analysis and judgement. The model includes decision making that can range from ill-structured decision making that relies on intuition, to well-structured decision making that incorporates information processing and analysis. The mode of decision making used will depend on the task in hand and the level and experience of the decision-maker.

An example of this would be where an experienced nurse on a surgical ward is caring for a patient who has undergone abdominal surgery. The patient appears restless, is a bit confused, looks pale and has shallow respirations.

- **Intuition:** the experienced surgical nurse will recognize that the appearance and behaviour of this patient suggest they may be bleeding. Only after they have recognized this will they check out their findings with the patient's observation chart and call the doctor.
- **Information processing and analysis:** as a student, you realize it is time to take the patient's observations. You check their temperature, pulse, respirations and blood pressure. You note that the pulse and respiratory rate have increased markedly. The blood pressure has fallen from 130/80 mmHg to 90/50 mmHg. You interpret the changes in the observations and decide to check the wound. The wound dressing is soaked in blood and the wound drain has drained a large amount since it was last checked. You use your knowledge of post-operative care to consider the findings, and realize you need to alert your mentor as soon as possible.

This example has demonstrated the two extremes of this decision making model. There will be variations in approach depending where you are on the continuum that the model describes. The crucial question that this book addresses is: where do you as a student nurse start with theories of decision making? What cognitive strategies and theories will you utilize as you progress through pre-registration courses to qualification? We propose the following framework as shown in Figure 1.2 to try and guide student nurses in their decision making.

The 'add on framework' of decision making

Years 1/2

In Figure 1.2 you will notice that Years 1/2 begin with the elements of information and reflection to incorporate into your decision making. You may gain information initially from previous employment and certainly from your early lectures, seminars, tutorials and background reading in your school of nursing course. You will be encouraged by your school of nursing to begin to reflect on the information you have received and to practise this in clinical placements. For instance, in clinical practice, you may have suggested a very simple decision to your mentor based on input you have previously had in your school of nursing. Your mentor may suggest that you reflect on your suggested decision; would any modification be appropriate in the light of clinical practice? You might realise that the information-processing model is at work here and this is often a feature of the novice decision-maker. The topic of reflection is considered later in Chapter 2.

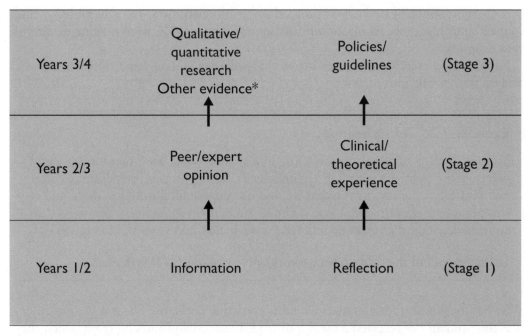

Years 3/4	Qualitative/ quantitative research Other evidence*	Policies/ guidelines	(Stage 3)
Years 2/3	Peer/expert opinion	Clinical/ theoretical experience	(Stage 2)
Years 1/2	Information	Reflection	(Stage 1)

Note: *This could comprise elements such as Cochrane Database Reviews, literature reviews, Department of Health and National Patient Safety Agency material.

Figure 1.2   The 'add on framework' for decision making

Years 2/3

Years 2/3 move a stage further in Figure 1.2. As you begin to move into different areas of practice, you will begin to take note of both peers (other students) perhaps from groupwork in theoretical sessions and your mentors. You may well come into contact with more specialist nurses such as community psychiatric nurses, key workers in learning disability settings, clinical nurse specialists who will influence your decision-making. Different clinical and theoretical experiences will begin to expand your ability to make decisions and you will begin to acquire more expertise moving towards an intuitive approach (probably via the cognitive continuum).

Years 3/4

Years 3/4 will see a move towards you beginning to take on board research and other evidence to support your decisions in practice. You will work more with policies and guidelines that are themselves based on best evidence and the decisions you make will become more sophisticated as you proceed towards registration. You will probably find yourself more and more taking an intuitive approach to your decision making in view of your experience.

Some simple exercises are given below that will give you an opportunity to put the 'add on framework' into practice.

Exercise 1.3 Adult branch

You are a junior student nurse working in a general ward. Your mentor has asked you to assist a patient with her hygiene needs. You approach the patient to offer her a wash but she says to you that she has not slept at all during the night and at this point feels very tired and would like to catch up on some sleep. You suggest to your mentor that the patient could have a wash later and your mentor agrees.

Using Stage 1 of the 'add on framework', give reasons for this decision.

Why has the junior student nurse made this particular decision? There is the possibility that this student has received some input from the school of nursing from which they will have learned that periods of sleep and rest are vital to aid recovery. The student might also have had from the same source some information on sleep deprivation. This has been reported in some quarters as leading to confusion, disorientation, low tolerance of pain and the possibility of poor tissue repair – although some studies regard the latter as controversial. It does demonstrate how initial information can influence decisions such as this. Reflecting and reviewing this decision, particularly with a mentor, can greatly influence future decision making. For instance, if the patient, after a period of sleep, demonstrated more energy and eagerness in carrying out hygiene needs, this decision could be said to be successful. If, however, after a period of sleep the patient was still tired and uninterested, the decision would not have been successful; there is a need to reflect and review further. Whatever the outcome, undertaking a review of the care decision (evaluation) will help. On reflection, future decision making might involve altering the timing of care interventions to set aside specific time periods for rest and sleep; does there need to be a review of analgesia administration to help promote sleep? Is there a case for introducing some complementary therapy to help promote sleep for such a patient? Out of such a simple decision, much can be learned for future clinical practice.

Exercise 1.4 Child branch

While undertaking your first clinical placement allocation on the paediatric ward, your mentor asks you to feed an 11-month-old infant, Noah. His mother, who has been resident during this admission, has gone home for a short period. Noah's assessment documentation states that he has a good appetite and that he is used to a diet with thicker/chunkier foods. You sit Noah in a high chair and offer him some pasta and mashed vegetables together with a yogurt for dessert and attempt to feed him. However, Noah keeps his lips tightly pursed and shakes his head as you attempt to spoon-feed him. You abandon attempting to feed him savoury food and endeavour to interest him in his 'favourite' food, yogurt. This time Noah rapidly becomes distressed and tearful. You decide that it is inappropriate to continue attempting to feed him and your mentor agrees.

Using Stage 1 of the 'add on framework', give reasons for this decision.

You will have received some information as to why maintaining an adequate nutritional status and documenting nutritional input is important for all clients. You may also have received some specific information pertaining to infants and weaning diets. Dependent on your experience of infants, you may have some knowledge of how difficult feeding children this age can be. At 11 months of age children will already have developed favourite foods and giving something slightly different may be enough to cause them to refuse food. In addition, Noah will also becoming more independent and may prefer feeding himself and refuse to be spoon-fed.

In a hospital situation it may just be that there is too much going on in the ward and Noah could be expressing his frustration that you have stopped him from exploring when you put him in the high chair. Likewise, it could be that because you are someone unfamiliar, he may refuse to eat until his Mum returns. It is important that you reflect on why you decided to give up feeding Noah at this time, including how you are going to document this information and how you may communicate this to Mum on her return and also whether you need to make a decision to attempt to feed again later on.

Exercise 1.5   Learning disability branch

You are a junior student working on an assessment and treatment unit. Your mentor asks you to help a service user go to the toilet.

When collecting the service user from the toilet, they say they didn't have any luck as it is 'too hard to come out'.

You decide to check the service user's records and realize that this person's bowels have not been opened for the last week.

What would your decision be in this situation? Use Stage 1 of the 'add on framework' to give reasons for your decision.

You may well have had some theoretical input with regard to elimination but this is likely to be limited. You need here to report the matter to your mentor who will advise you (in the light of his or her practical experience) about what should be done about this situation. There could be a number of measures to be taken here to resolve the situation. These measures may vary from medication, dietary elements and increased mobilization, but it is important that you think about such situations and learn from these. Learning from these experiences includes thinking about and finding out how such problems could be prevented in the future.

Now consider a student nurse in a later stage of his or her course. An additional tier of the 'add on framework' could operate here.

Exercise 1.6 Adult branch

You are a student nurse who is in the second half of the second year of the course. You are working in a health care of the elderly ward and are asked to get a patient out of bed for breakfast. The patient has already had his medication half an hour ago. You help the patient to sit up on the side of his bed but you are uncertain of his ability to stand up at this point. You decide to let the patient sit on the side of the bed for five minutes in order that you are satisfied that he can stand safely and transfer to the chair.

What might have led you to make this decision? Use Stage 2 of the 'add on framework' to help.

You will have had information on safe handling of patients and also circulatory disorders. On previous clinical experience, you might have seen patients not transfer successfully if the manoeuvre is attempted too quickly. During a medication administration round, this patient might have received drugs for hypertension. Previous discussion with peers and mentors from their experience and practice may have identified similar problems and how to deal with them successfully.

Exercise 1.7 Learning disabilities

George has just had a tonic clonic seizure. He is obviously confused and is trying to get out of the chair. When he stands up he is obviously unstable. You encourage him to go and rest in his bed.

What might have led you to make this decision? Use Stage 2 of the 'add on framework' to help.

Exercise 1.8   Mental health

Henry Uppingham is an 82-year-old man resident on a unit for the care of the older person. He suffers from fluctuating periods of confusion and restlessness that tend to be worse in the early hours of the morning. Prior to retirement, he worked as a milkman. During these periods of confusion, he gets out of bed and becomes very restless and resistant insisting that he must get to work or he will be late.

During the day, Henry is moderately confused but responds well to verbal prompting and encouragement. Staff that have nursed Henry for a while recognize that when he needs to go to the toilet he becomes more restless and paces the ward. In these situations, Henry responds well to verbal prompting and simple directions to the toilet. He walks well with the assistance of one nurse but requires a wheelchair for long journeys.

Although with the support of staff Henry can mostly find his way around the familiar environment of the ward, he quickly becomes disoriented in unfamiliar settings, which adds to his increasing confusion and anxiety. Henry has formed a positive therapeutic relationship with a junior student on the ward called Jenny.

It is decided to take five residents of the ward for a cream tea at the local fête. Discussions are being held whether to include Henry in the trip or not.

? What factors might influence the decision to include Henry in the trip or not?

? What might be the implications of including Henry in this trip?

? What other decisions would need to be considered to ensure a successful conclusion to the trip?

Use Stage 2 of the 'add on framework' to help.

You will have received relevant theoretical input on the safe administration of medications as well as information pertaining to the importance of maintaining body temperature, the role of antipyretics and importance of gaining consent and cooperation. On previous clinical placements, you may have seen children and young people refuse medication and may have identified strategies as to how to manage each individual situation. This may include exploring alternate methods of administration of paracetamol other than via the oral administration route as well as considering whether other methods of reducing body temperature would be appropriate.

Consider now the later stage of the course (third or fourth year) and examine the situation when the framework in its entirety is applied

Exercise 1.9

Adult Branch

You are a third-year student nurse and are in your final placement on a ward specializing in circulatory disorders. A patient is admitted from home with a sacral pressure sore. From your assessment of the sore, you note that infection is present. A wound swab is taken and when results are available, you consult the ward formulary for wound-dressing products and note that it had been compiled a number of years ago. In a previous community experience, you have utilized Acquacel[Ag] (Dowsett, 2004) for an identical situation. Even though this is not in the wound formulary, you feel this type of dressing would be the most effective in this case. The ward manager agrees in the light of your justification and evidence and a supply of the wound product is obtained. (As a follow-up to this incident, the ward manager contacts the responsible authority for updating of the wound formulary.)

Learning Disabilities

Linda, who has multiple disabilities has just been discharged from an acute NHS hospital to her home. You are a student currently working in a community learning disability team. Your mentor receives a referral about Linda. Linda's mother and father have just returned from a holiday (they took the opportunity to have a few days away while she was in hospital) and are concerned as she has returned from hospital emaciated, lethargic, she has a dry mouth and her skin is not in a very good condition.

Note: It may be useful to refer to *Death by Indifference* (MENCAP, 2007).

Child Branch

You are undertaking a year three placement allocation on a general paediatric ward in a district general hospital. A 13-year-old young person has been admitted as an emergency following a road traffic accident. The young person has sustained a fractured right tibia and is under the care of the adult orthopaedic surgeons. The orthopaedic surgeon advises that the young person will be unable to be taken to theatre until the following day when he will be added to the end of the morning theatre list. Nevertheless, the surgeon requests that the young person is to be fasted in preparation for surgery; that is, Nil By Mouth (NBM) from midnight. You are aware that this contravenes both contemporary evidence and the local paediatric policy for preoperative patients and advise the surgeon accordingly. The surgeon repeats the instruction for the young person to be NBM from midnight and immediately leaves the ward. Consequently, you alert the ward manager and anaesthetist of the instructions, and as a result of your actions the young person will be able to have a light early breakfast at 06.00 and clear fluids until 08.00 when he will become NBM.

In applying Stage 3 of the 'add on framework' you will appreciate how research and experience play a part in your decision making. Wound care has been the subject of much nursing research and an area in which the nursing profession has now acquired much expertise. A word of caution – nurses need to be able to appraise research effectively; careful thought and deliberation are required before incorporating research into practice. We discuss this more in Chapter 3 related to using evidence in practice.

However, as you progress through your pre-registration course, you will be aware of how the components of the 'add on framework' influence your decision making.

What can constrain or promote decision making?

Earlier in the chapter, the role of the nurse was highlighted as becoming more complex than ever. The issues of governmental reforms and initiatives were also mentioned. It is important that any discussion of decision making takes these elements into account. They may be seen as both constraining and promoting decision making.

What might constrain effective decision making?

Nurses must act constantly in the best interests of their patients. The NMC (2008: 7) Code specifies this as follows: 'Provide a high standard of practice and care at all time.' This means that effective clinical decisions must be made in order to ensure the best outcome for patients. However, constraints exist that can impact on decision making. Examples of these are outlined below.

Resources (where these are inadequate or unsuitable)

The nurse may experience problems when wanting to make decisions in the best interests of patients. These can include a poor skill mix where there is an inadequate number of experienced staff to carry out care; hotel services where these are poorly organized and might result in a reduced availability of suitable food for patients; poor environmental facilities such as lack of suitable storage space for equipment compromises the safety of all parties.

Organizational objectives

There is no doubt that organizational objectives can also constrain decision making – consider the situation from a prevention of infection perspective. A Department of Health (2007) report found a relationship between bed occupancy and MRSA rates. In the period 2001–2004, trusts running at bed occupancy of 90 per cent had MRSA rates more than 10 per cent higher than those below 85 per cent. Curiously, in the period 2004–2006, the rates of infection were broadly similar irrespective of bed occupancy.

For example, in an effort to meet waiting time targets, a patient may experience one, two or even three transfers between hospital wards – often at short notice – this may not allow time for necessary decontamination of equipment between patients, leading to the spread of infection. A third-year nurse in a final management clinical placement will become acutely aware of this while working in such a setting.

What might promote decision making?

As you are undertaking a pre-registration nursing course, you will need ultimately to be able to manage the care for a number of patients. While you are a student, you will always have a mentor/supervisor who will sanction your decisions, or not as the case may be. While you can expect some supervisory help in the early stages after the point of qualification, there will come a point where you will have to make decisions for yourself. As nurses, we cover the 24-hour cycle of care – this means that there will be periods where nurses alone are present in care areas and this is a very powerful promoter for decision making, particularly at night. Think of the situation where you are faced with the dilemma with no medical back-up near at hand; do you call out the doctor or not? In such a case, you *will* be asked to justify your decision. If you have had previous experiences of such a situation, you will be more confident in the decision that you make. Therefore, as students, it is necessary to have relevant clinical experiences that do cover the 24-hour cycle of care.

Nursing is constantly widening the boundaries of practice. This element will involve even more decision making, often at a very high level. Think of the remit of the community psychiatric nurse or the diabetes specialist nurse and the types of decision that they may make. The profession will expect us in the future to make even more sophisticated decisions as aspects of care change and new developments occur.

Conclusion

The 'add on framework' can help a student to gain the best from a nursing course and clinical experience. It is also important to seek out learning opportunities in each placement. Use reflection from an early stage. Use your experience/portfolio to inform future practice. Utilize specialist services and, where possible, other professions to inform practice. Learn the art of critically appraising evidence including a very serious consideration of: 'Is this credible for *my* practice?' Most of all, listen and try to act on what your patients say to you!

References

Cader, R., Campbell, S. and Watson, D. (2005) Cognitive continuum theory in nursing decision-making, *Journal of Advanced Nursing*, 49(4): 397–405.

Department of Health (DoH) (2007) *Hospital Organisation, Speciality Mix and MRSA*. London: DoH.

Dowsett, C. (2004) The use of silver-based dressings in wound care, *Nursing Standard*, 19(7): 55–60.

Mencap (2007) *Death by Indifference*. London: Mencap.

Muir, N. (2004) Clinical decision making: theory and practice, *Nursing Standard*, 18(36): 45–52.

Nursing and Midwifery Council (NMC) (2008) *The Code: Standards of Conduct, Performance and Ethics for Nurses and Midwives*. London: NMC.

Nursing and Midwifery Council (NMC) (2009) *Guidance on Professional Conduct for Nursing and Midwifery Students*. London: NMC.

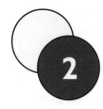

2 Using professional skills to support decision making: using reflection to learn from experience

- **Introduction**
- **What is nursing?**
- **A skills escalator approach to nursing**
- **The 'add on framework' for decision making**
- **Reflection in nursing: how this helps us to make decisions**
- **Models of reflection**
- **Conclusion**
- **References**
- **Further reading**

Introduction

In Chapter 1 we explored making decisions in a professional capacity, theories of decision making and levels of decision making. In this chapter we explore how to use professional skills as a nurse to support your decisions. This includes being able to define nursing and have a clear understanding of the parameters you need to work within to make good decisions. In making decisions it is important to be able to define nursing in order to know the parameters you need to work within in order to be able to make your decisions. In addition, we explore the importance of reflection and how reflection can help us to clarify why we make certain decisions, as well as how we can learn from the decisions that we make in order to influence and refine our future practice. The process of learning from experience helps us to develop an awareness of how we can use professional reasoning to inform the decisions that we make. We also show you how we can use a skills escalator approach in order to be aware of what is expected of you at specific levels within the education programme in terms of the practice of nursing, including the increasingly complex reasoning skills necessary to function at particular levels.

What is nursing?

Defining nursing is difficult and there is no legal definition of nursing in the United Kingdom (UK), even though nursing is experienced by everyone at some time in their life. We may all be 'nursed' by someone who is not part of the nursing profession; for example, babies and children are often nursed by their parents when they are ill but this does not mean that the person caring for their child is a nurse in the professional sense. This is why it is important for nurses in a professional capacity to have a definition of what they provide that a layperson who is nursing someone does not provide. In fact, in the *Concise Oxford Dictionary*, the term 'definition' means 'the formal statement of the meaning of a word, phrase ...'. However, many definitions of nursing are available within the literature that originate from various sources both within and outside of the UK some of which we explore later.

When you first thought of becoming a nurse you must have formed an idea of what nursing was in order to help you make this choice of career. Think back to when you first thought of or started nursing, what did you think nursing entailed?

Exercise 2.1

I thought that nursing was ...

You may have included some or all of the following:

- You wanted to work with people.
- You wanted to care for people.
- You respected nurses and wanted to be like them.
- You wanted to learn about the body.
- You wanted to feel needed.
- You wanted to contribute something to society.
- You wanted to make a difference to people.

Of course, you may have thought of other things. What is important is, have your ideas and understanding of nursing changed since you have worked in a professional setting? From your experiences in nursing, what would your own definition of nursing be at this point?

Exercise 2.2

I now believe that nursing is …

Think about how easy or difficult it was to describe what you believe nursing to be. If you found defining nursing difficult, you would not be alone.

My own personal definition is that caring is central to nursing combined with the relevant knowledge, technical skills, interpersonal approaches and professional behaviours combined in such a way as to make the patient central to the process of nursing. The nurse will demonstrate the ability to 'be' with the patient in helping the patient to make informed choices in the situation in which they find themselves. Throughout these processes, the nurse will make decisions both for and with the patient at various times depending on the patient situation, while working alongside other health care professionals and taking into account their perspectives on the patient's care.

This definition has taken me a long time to develop and I have probably been influenced by other writers, my colleagues' beliefs, and by my own development within the nursing profession.

Virginia Henderson (cited in RCN, 2000: 6) defines nursing as 'to assist the individual, sick or well, in the performance of those activities contributing to health or its recovery (or to peaceful death) that the individual would perform unaided if he had the necessary strength, will or knowledge'. Henderson also goes on to talk about how the nurse works independently on some aspects of the nursing role but also how the nurse is part of a team, helping medical staff to implement treatment for patients. Henderson describes aspects of nursing that are solely the role and function of the nurse but also describes how nurses work with and for other professionals; hence, communication is a key element of nursing.

More recently, the RCN (2000: 3) has defined nursing as 'the use of clinical judgement in the provision of care to enable people to improve, maintain or recover health to cope with health problems and to achieve the best possible quality of life whatever their disease or disability, until death'. As can be seen from the RCN description, decision making and clinical judgement feature strongly and so it is imperative that students work towards achieving good decision making skills. In fact, the core difference between a health care support worker and a registered nurse is that of the nurse being able to make clinical decisions about care using sound clinical judgement. The RCN (2000) goes on to describe how professional nursing incorporates knowledge, personal accountability for all decisions and actions, as well as a structured relationship between the nurse and patient that incorporates professional regulation and a code of ethics within a statutory framework.

Defining what nursing is enables the public to have an understanding of what can be expected from nurses. This is extremely important when building a structured relationship with patients in order for all parties to have realistic expectations of what the nurse is able to provide. Part of the problem in defining nursing is that the many and varied generic and specialist roles that nurses take on can confuse core definitions of what nursing is and should be for all its patients/clients.

Midwifery definitions are much more focused and are described as 'health professionals who provide primary care to women and their babies during pregnancy, labour, birth and the postpartum period' (Canadian Association of Midwives, 2009). However, this definition does not acknowledge the support role of the family as a whole, that is, the family dynamics that have to be taken into account during these periods of care. In addition, it does not encapsulate the many roles that the midwife has to become proficient in within its brief definition.

Whatever definition of nursing or midwifery that you adopt or create, as professionals we must be able to communicate our beliefs about what nursing is in order to enhance the public's understanding of what we do. A universal definition of nursing/midwifery would help in this, and would help us to articulate what nurses, in particular, do. Some of the further reading at the end of this chapter will be useful in helping you to evaluate what nursing/midwifery is.

In defining nursing and midwifery, a statement is being made about what is central to the professions and hence what the public/patients will expect us to make decisions about.

What nursing and midwifery do include are the following:

- knowledge
- technical expertise
- communication
- interpersonal approaches
- social and emotional care
- caring
- meeting patient's needs whether empowering individuals, facilitating care, promoting independence or delivering care
- promotion of health
- maintenance of health
- teaching
- teamwork
- managing care.

In undertaking nursing and midwifery, some or all of the above may be utilized within a given situation to influence the decisions that we make. What complicates defining nursing further is that there are different branches of nursing in which the emphasis of specific aspects of nursing will vary, as well as differing specialties within each branch of nursing that influence the types of decision about nursing that the individual is empowered to make.

However, if you consider the aspects that nursing does include, it can be seen to be complex, taking into account many factors in order to use clinical reasoning in order to make decisions about care, either with or for the individual.

Read through the following vignettes and complete Exercise 2.3.

Exercise 2.3

Learning disability nursing

Sarah is a 16-year-old who has cerebral palsy who attends a day centre. She has some difficulty in walking and with her speech but is able to live at home. She is very conscious of her mobility problems and her speech. She becomes upset and frustrated as she wants to join in with the activities her two teenage sisters enjoy. However, she also lacks confidence as she doesn't cope well with meeting new people.

Adult nursing

Mr Brown is 40 years old, married and has two teenage children. He has bowel cancer that has spread to his liver and spine. He has a colostomy to relieve the bowel obstruction. He is also weak and unsteady on his feet. He understands there is no cure and wants to go home to make the most of the time left to him. His wife and children are devastated at the possibility of losing him.

Mental health nursing

Alex is a 22-year-old who is suffering from depression and anxiety. He normally works as a retail assistant in a large department store but is off sick currently. His girlfriend of six years has recently left him for someone else. He was devastated as they were planning to get married. Shortly after the break-up he lost both his maternal grandparents who he was very close to. He feels he is a failure in life. He lacks interest in himself, his physical appearance and friends. He is also quite withdrawn.

Children's nursing

Sally is nearly 4 years old and has recently been diagnosed with asthma. She has had an acute admission to the paediatric unit for severe breathing difficulties. Her mother is anxious about Sally's condition and her ability to cope with it. An additional concern for her mother is that Sally is due to start school soon.

Midwifery

At an antenatal booking clinic while obtaining a history from the expectant mother, the midwife discovers that the mother is a heavy smoker. The expectant mother, due to her adverse domestic circumstances, appears unwilling to consider stopping smoking.

Consider these vignettes from across the branches of nursing and midwifery:

 What sort of interventions might be required for each individual?

 What might the aims be for each patient/service user?

 How does the type of nursing/midwifery intervention differ for each branch, and how is it similar?

A skills escalator approach to nursing

Having looked at what nursing is, we need to explore the different levels of practice you need to work towards, which will inevitably affect your ability to make decisions about care.

Bondy (1983) describes a skills escalator approach to identify the level of practice expected to be achieved at specific points when developing nursing expertise. This skills escalator describes four practice levels as can be seen from Figure 2.1. We have adapted Bondy's work to incorporate the practice levels that could be expected at specific points within the pre-registration programmes.

The arrows in Figure 2.1 show how a student who is experiencing different types of placement experience might move up and down the skills escalator. For example, a student who has worked within an acute elderly care placement may have achieved the ability to only need assistance from time to time from their mentor (Bondy practice Level 2) but when they move to an intensive care unit setting, they may move back to requiring constant supervision (Bondy Level 1). This does not mean that the student has regressed in terms of their nursing expertise, only that the type of nursing being experienced is unfamiliar, needing different skills and knowledge that the student has to learn in order to be safe in delivering care in this type of setting. However, as can be seen from Figure 2.1, the student must achieve a minimum level at specific points in their course.

Bondy (1983) describes what is required for differing levels of practice in a skills escalator.

Practice Achievement Level for Students
(Adapted from Bondy's Skills Escalator)

A skills escalator means that students can move up and down levels of achievement, depending on the student and the type of placement; for example, the student's level of achievement in a social care setting may differ from their achievement in a critical setting or community setting. What is important is that the student is given credit for their performance. However, all students must achieve the minimum of specific points in the course.

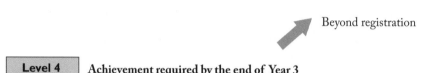

Beyond registration

Level 4   Achievement required by the end of Year 3

This means:

- practises with minimal supervision, in accordance with NMC and local trust requirements, meeting the standards of proficiency
- seeks advice and support, as appropriate.
- demonstrates knowledge, skills and attitude appropriate to this level.

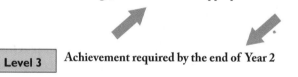

Level 3   Achievement required by the end of Year 2

This means:

- practises with decreasing supervision
- requires occasional support and prompts in the development of appropriate knowledge, skills and attitudes.

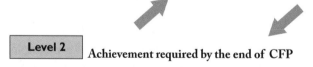

Level 2   Achievement required by the end of CFP

Practises with assistance in the delivery of care to achieve practice outcomes. Demonstrates knowledge, skills and attitudes to achieve this level.

Level I

Student practises with constant supervision in the delivery of essential care to develop the knowledge, skills and attitude required to achieve practice outcomes.

Figure 2.1   The skills escalator

Level 1: the student should be able to practise safely and professionally under constant supervision. In addition, the student should begin to be able to identify where information may be accessed in order to support their practice. For example, the student should be aware of where local policies and procedures are located in order to begin to learn about how and why care is delivered in a particular way. In addition, they should demonstrate that they are developing good communication skills. For example, you can help a patient to have a wash with your mentor after you have accessed and read the local procedure about infection control issues when meeting a patient's hygiene needs. In addition, you demonstrate to your mentor that you can help to make the patient feel relaxed by talking to them about their family and home life.

Level 2: the student should now be able to apply theoretical knowledge to clinical practice that can help them to make judgements about care. These judgements might involve beginning to prioritize care and adapt care under fairly close supervision. Effective communication should be demonstrated when interacting with patients and the nursing team. For example, when taking a patient's observations post-operatively, you note that their pulse rate has increased from 80 beats per minute to 96, their blood pressure has fallen from 120/80 to 110/60, and their respirations have increased from 16 per minute to 24. You know from reading about post-operative care that the patient may be going into shock. You check their wound drainage system and note a large amount of blood has drained. You decide you need to alert your mentor straight away as this patient may be bleeding.

Level 3: at this level the student should start to develop increasing independence in initiating actions. They should also be able to start to critically evaluate evidence and be able to use evidence to make informed judgements about care delivery. Communication skills should be developing in effectiveness with nursing and health/social care professionals. For example, you ask a child who appears to be in pain in an in-patient setting how he is today. He tells you he has diarrhoea. You find out that he has had severe diarrhoea all night, abdominal cramps and he feels feverish. You decide to ask your mentor if it is alright to take a stool specimen, put the patient on a stool chart, move the patient into a single room, and increase the frequency of their vital sign observations. You are aware of local infection control procedures, the risk to this child's health, know that other patients in the area are immunosuppressed and that, if the diarrhoea has an infectious cause, this could be catastrophic for other patients who are already ill.

Level 4: the student needs to demonstrate they are moving towards independent practice. They should be able to draw on a wide range of resources, using sound, evidence-based rationales for their decisions. In addition, they should be able to consistently communicate effectively with a variety of health care professionals. An example of a Level 4 decision might be that while admitting a patient and undertaking a pressure risk assessment, you identify this patient to be at high risk of developing a pressure sore as they are undernourished, immobile and on bedrest, and in severe pain.

You utilize the risk assessment procedure to identify the patient requires a pressure-relieving mattress, call the equipment service department and order a pressure-relieving mattress for this patient, and document your actions. You inform your mentor of your actions, ask her to countersign your care plan entry, and ask if there is anything else that your mentor feels needs to be done.

Using the four levels of practice on Bondy's skills escalator, consider the following scenarios in Exercises 2.4 and 2.5 that focuses on how Bondy's practice levels can be achieved:

Exercise 2.4   Adult branch

You are helping Mrs Brown to sit out in a chair and ask her if she has had a good night's sleep if she is ready for her breakfast. She tells you she has been up to the toilet all night and feels pretty awful. She also says it is a bit uncomfortable when she passes urine.

Using Table 2.1, consider this brief scenario and try to identify what might be required of you at each practice level of Bondy in terms of this patient. *Note*: How much of this you can complete will depend on the level you are at within your own course currently.

Bondy practice Level 1	Bondy practice Level 2	Bondy practice Level 3	Bondy practice Level 4

Table 2.1   Using Bondy's skills escalator

Table 2.2 demonstrates the practice required for each level of practice, adult branch, according to Bondy, for example,

- At practice Level 1, you are alerted to a problem and make a decision to tell your mentor. The mentor then decides how to proceed with your help.
- For practice Level 2, having learned from previous experience, you make the decision to elicit more information, can make the decision to undertake some investigations (urine testing), decide to document results and then go to your mentor with more information about Mrs Brown's problem.
- At practice Level 3, you build on Level 2 by making links and suggesting actions that will help to clarify what Mrs Brown's problem is.
- At practice Level 4, you utilize more sophisticated decision making skills in terms of patient observation, obtaining more information and initiating actions while still clarifying with your mentor that your decisions are appropriate.

These scenarios demonstrate how the Bondy skills escalator can be applied to your sphere of practice. It also identifies the level of practice expected from you as you proceed on your nursing/midwifery programme. The Bondy levels can also be linked to the 'add on framework' for decision making. If you remember from Chapter 1, there are three stages:

- **Stage 1 (initial influences):** you start to gather information and reflect on the experiences you have had.
- **Stage 2 (using evidence):** you learn from peers and experts you work with, using theoretical and clinical evidence to make decisions
- **Stage 3 (using research):** you can utilize both research and policies/guidelines that you have critically evaluated to inform the decisions you make.

Consider Exercise 2.5 in which you have identified the Bondy practice levels and which actions might be incorporated into each level. Think about what decisions were made.

Table 2.3 demonstrates the practice required for each level of practice, child branch.

Exercise 2.5   Child branch

Sally Lewis, aged 4, has recently been diagnosed as suffering from asthma. She has had an acute admission to the paediatric ward for a severe exacerbation of her asthma and has been commenced on an inhaler via a spacer and facemask. While administering Sally's inhaler, her mother states that she is quite anxious about Sally's recent diagnosis and her ability to cope with the situation. An additional concern is that Sally is shortly to commence school.

Practice Level 1	You inform your mentor of what Mrs Brown has said
	Your mentor asks you to take Mrs Brown's temperature
	The mentor supervises you testing her urine and charting the results
	The mentor shows you how to document Mrs Brown's problem and the observations obtained in the plan of care
Practice Level 2	You ask Mrs Brown if passing urine causes a burning sensation and how long she has had this and what the discomfort is like
	You test the urine of Mrs Brown and note the colour and smell, and chart the results
	You inform your mentor of your findings, document your findings and get your mentor to countersign the entry in the plan of care
	Your mentor prompts you to take the patient's temperature and inform her of the result after documenting the result
Practice Level 3	You undertake all the practice Level 2 actions and ask Mrs Brown how much she has been drinking
	When reporting to your mentor you ask if a midstream specimen of urine needs to be obtained for culture and sensitivity, and ask the doctor to write a request form
	You obtain the midstream specimen and send it to the laboratory
	Your also ask your mentor if you can do a bladder scan to see if there is a residual urine as you have been reading about how useful this can be in helping to contribute to a urinary assessment of a patient
	You document all actions and ask your mentor to countersign your entry in the plan of care
Practice Level 4	You notice Mrs Brown looks tired, unwell and in some discomfort before you ask some prompting questions as to why
	You undertake all the previous actions, but still consult your mentor as to whether a bladder scan to ascertain the residual urine is needed
	You consult with your mentor to see if a fluid balance chart is appropriate as you note Mrs Brown has a dry mouth, her skin is inelastic and you are worried she may not be drinking much
	You note from the patient's history that she has had several urinary tract infections over the last year and consult with the mentor and medical staff to gain permission to start Mrs Brown on cranberry juice as you are aware from a Cochrane review (Jepson, 2007) that there is sound evidence that cranberry juice may decrease the number of urinary symptomatic infections
	You document all actions and findings, asking your mentor to countersign your entry in the plan of care

Table 2.2 Practice required for each level of Bondy – adult branch

Practice Level 1	The mentor demonstrates how to administer Sally's inhaler and you both document it on the prescription chart.
	You inform your mentor of what Mrs Lewis has said. The mentor asks you to play with Sally to distract her while she talks to Mrs Lewis to see what her concerns are.
	The mentor shows you how to document Mrs Lewis's concerns in the care plan and shows you how to refer Sally to the respiratory nurse and school nursing service so she has support after discharge.
Practice Level 2	The mentor supervises you administering Sally's inhaler and you document administration together.
	You ask Mrs Lewis what her anxieties are about coping with Sally's asthma. She feels she won't be able to cope with using the inhaler and spacer device. She is anxious about recognising deterioration in Sally's condition and whether Sally will cope at school. You inform the mentor of your discussion, document the issues and get your mentor to countersign it in the care plan.
	Your mentor prompts you to refer Sally to the respiratory nurse and school nursing services. You inform Mrs Lewis of your actions.
Practice Level 3	You undertake all actions at Level 2.
	You ask your mentor if you can provide some written information about asthma for Sally and her mum.
	You ask your mentor if you can start an education programme with Sally's mum to teach her about inhaler technique as you are aware from the literature that inhaler techniques are often poor.
	You ask if it is appropriate to initiate a referral to the school nursing service so that Sally can be assessed in school.
	You document all actions and ask the mentor to countersign them.
Practice Level 4	You undertake all the previous actions.
	You observe that Sally has picked up her mum's anxieties and she is getting upset about taking her inhaler. You consult with your mentor and Mrs Lewis to ask if you can involve the play specialist as you know that therapeutic play can help young children to overcome anxieties associated with therapies and this can increase compliance with therapy.
	You note that Mrs Lewis frequently leaves the ward to go for a cigarette. You know that parental smoking has an impact on a child's asthma and the severity of symptoms. You ask your mentor and the doctor if it might be appropriate to refer Mrs Lewis for some support to stop smoking. You also give Mrs Lewis the details of support groups to help people to stop smoking.
	You document all actions and ask your mentor to countersign your entry in the care plan.

Table 2.3   Practice required for each level of Bondy – child branch

Exercise 2.6

Which stages within the 'add on framework' for decision making do these scenario decisions fit into?

Stage 1	Stage 2	Stage 3

The 'add on framework' for decision making

Relating back to the adult scenario in Exercise 2.4, we can explore the stages of decision making.

Stage 1 (initial influences)

The student recognizes there might be a problem for this patient and decides to inform the mentor. If the mentor had not been informed (a decision in itself), the patient's condition might not have been recognized and treatment might have been delayed resulting in further discomfort for the patient/child and the potential for the individual's condition to deteriorate.

Stages 1–2 (initial influences and some clinical experience)

The nurse begins to use her past experience and decides to ask more specific questions to ascertain more information before deciding to report it to the mentor. In addition, the student decides to test the urine so that the mentor has more information to base her judgement on.

Stage 2 (initial influences, past experience and theoretical knowledge)

You make a decision to test the urine, start to utilize your knowledge and past experience as you know that the presence of nitrites in the urine indicates a urine infection. You are also making a tentative decision to send a midstream urine sample by checking with your mentor if that is all right to do. You are also aware at this stage that a reduced fluid intake can make the elderly more prone to urinary tract infections. You also start to select from various options available to you, for example, ask about scanning the bladder using knowledge gained from reading around this topic.

Stage 3 (later influences)

Later influences play a significant part in your decision making as you utilize your observational skills, previous experiences, theoretical knowledge and research. You make several decisions at this stage that contribute to a structured plan for dealing with this person's problem. You decide to:

- ask prompting questions based on your observation of the patient, their initial responses and your previous experience
- initiate a plan of action to test the urine and, based on your findings, decide to send a midstream urine sample
- suggest to the mentor the need to obtain a residual urine as there may be other problems with bladder emptying that may have contributed to the development of a urinary tract infection
- suggest monitoring the patient's fluid intake and output based on the observations you make on the patient
- make a decision to consult previous patient records to ascertain if the patient has a history that is relevant to this situation
- utilize research to help make the decision to administer cranberry juice to the patient when consulting with your mentor and the medical staff
- make a decision regarding the relevant details that need to be recorded in the patient's documentation.

This simple scenario demonstrates how, as a student progresses, the decisions that are made about a patient's care become increasingly complex and how increasing responsibility as a student contributes to the level of decision making required when working towards becoming a registered nurse.

The decisions we make are based on:

- recognition of an issue/problem
- using previous experience to decide on actions
- seeking advice from other personnel
- using evidence to support and inform your actions
- selecting actions from available options
- knowing when to alert other health care professionals to issues/problems
- acknowledging own limitations.

Exercise 2.7

Using an example from your own practice, think about your experience and:

- describe how you responded to a situation
- the decision/s that you made
- where the decisions fit on the 'add on framework'
- how you might improve your level of decision making.

It will also be useful to think about what knowledge or skills might help you to develop in relation to similar scenarios in the future.

Description	Decisions made	Stage on the 'add on framework'	Future learning

From your examples it should now be clear that we need to learn from our experiences in order to become competent professionals who are providing expert care for our patients based on the best available evidence. However, just because we have experience of something does not mean we learn and develop from our experience. Within our lives we probably all know someone (maybe even ourselves) who tends to make the same mistake over and over again. Hence, we have to work at developing our learning about the art and science of nursing in a structured way, and reflective practice is a way of helping us to learn and develop from our experiences.

Reflection in nursing: how this helps us to make decisions

Within the nursing environment the decisions we make affect the (often) vulnerable individuals that we are caring for. Therefore, it is important to ensure that we learn from our experience and learn how to develop our skills, knowledge and expertise in order to become a skilled practitioner of nursing. Reflection is a useful way to use our experience and learn from it. How reflection is structured is very much an individual preference and much has been published about reflection and how a framework can be used within the reflective process in order to learn and develop in a structured way.

Nurses who are practising today are required to anticipate and manage patients in a highly complex and uncertain health care environment (Candela et al., 2008). As a student nurse you are working towards this goal in order to be able to function as a newly registered nurse. Working towards being able to do this requires you, as a student, to move from being a passive receiver of information to being an independent, self-directed, active nurse who bases their care on the best available evidence.

Nurses today must possess high-level reasoning skills to deal with complex patient care and the sort of problems that nurses frequently encounter in the practice setting (Murphy, 2004). Reflection can assist the development of reasoning skills helping the nurse to become someone who is able to generate, implement and evaluate approaches to care as he or she moves from being a novice in nursing towards becoming an expert. As a student this might sound unattainable at this point but this is the goal you need to work towards. Within the profession we have all started out as novices and the challenge in becoming part of the nursing profession is to work towards becoming an expert practitioner. This is not something that happens accidentally. Becoming an expert needs to be worked at in order for us to develop complex clinical reasoning that will assist us in developing decision making skills. In working at this we should be able to provide expert nursing for the individuals we are providing care for. Reflection can help us to develop these skills. Murphy (2004) found in her research that students who were higher clinical reasoners reported a higher frequency of the use of focused reflection and articulation to promote clinical reasoning. Hence, it follows that in developing our use of reflection, we can develop our clinical reasoning and ability to make effective and appropriate decisions with and for patients.

Reflection is a process that can be used to assist with learning. It can both inform and improve practice (Parsons and White, 2007). As a student your learning curve is steep, and reflection can help you to integrate what is taught in the classroom with what is experienced in clinical practice (Nicholl and Higgins, 2004). It can also inspire you to build on your existing knowledge (Clements, 2007).

Reflection is a process of reviewing practice experience in order to describe, analyse, evaluate and so inform learning about practice (Reid, 1993). Atkins in Burns and Bulman (2000) outlines several underlying skills that are required for reflective practice (this is summarized in Table 2.4).

Self-awareness	This underpins the entire process of reflection. It requires honesty and enables analysis of situations. Honesty can sometimes be somewhat painful as you might feel you haven't coped particularly well during this example of your experience. For example, you are present at a cardiac arrest and feel very upset that you panicked and didn't feel you were any help as you forgot all the training you had received
Description	There is a need to be able to describe key elements of your experience accurately in order to be able to analyse experiences. For example, this is the first cardiac arrest you have been present at. You checked the patient for the presence of respirations and a pulse. Both were absent. At this point you shouted for someone to come rather than using the emergency call system. You had to be asked to fetch the arrest trolley, and couldn't remember how to perform chest compressions
Critical analysis	This is about separating out the whole experience into component parts. It allows a detailed examination of these component parts (analysis) that enables you to make judgements about the strengths and weaknesses of component parts. This part of the process allows you to also explore your feelings, identify your assumptions, challenge your assumptions, and identify and explore alternative courses of action. For example, in this instance you realize you panicked but this was the first time you had seen an arrest. You are aware you shied away from practising resuscitation in front of your peers in the classroom and so didn't feel as competent as you might have. However, you were able to check for breathing and the absence of a pulse and did know to get someone immediately. You also realize you need to ask for some more resuscitation practice in the university, need to ask your mentor to go through the arrest trolley with you, and that you need to practise this skill until you can do it without thinking about it
Synthesis	This is the skill that allows you to build up the experience into a coherent whole, integrating new knowledge, skills, feelings and attitudes You have learned that you need to develop more confidence in the classroom, be more proactive when participating in clinical skills sessions so that you feel more confident about your ability in the future. You also identify your need to attend the university assertiveness course to help you gain more confidence in your ability to deal with situations
Evaluation	Evaluation ensures that you review the learning that has taken place and what may still be required in order for you to develop your learning to a new level. For example, although you haven't encountered another cardiac arrest, you feel you will be able to cope better now you have gained more practice in the university. With the help of your mentor, you can now identify what each piece of equipment on the arrest trolley is for. You ask your mentor if you can attend a resuscitation session that the staff go to within the placement area you are working

Table 2.4 Skills of reflective practice

Exercise 2.8

Think about these underlying skills required for reflection. How have you, or how will you work at developing these skills?

Models of reflection

Schön (1983) also describes the ability to reflect *in* action and *on* action. However, for the purpose of this chapter, we are going to concentrate on reflection *on* action, using Driscoll's (1994), model which is a simple model that is easy to remember. It focuses on three stages: what?, so what? and now what?

❶ **What?** A description of an event in which you purposely reflect on aspects of that experience.
❷ **So what?** This is an analysis of the event from a personal, emotional, professional and/or a developmental perspective.
❸ **Now what?** Actioning the learning from that experience. Asking questions such as, where could you obtain the knowledge or skills that you need to face similar situations? Is action required at a personal, professional or organizational level? Implementing what you have learned in your future practice.

The following example in Table 2.5 may help you to understand the use of reflection in learning.

Reflection is an essential skill as it helps you to understand the world around you, and often to identify how things might be improved or carried out more effectively in the future (Williamson et al., 2008). In a complex ever changing environment in health care, nurses need skills to be able to continually develop their practice.

In order to undertake reflection, there are a set of skills you need to learn how to use. Like any skill such as learning how to drive, they have to be practised in order for you to become fluid and competent at them. At first you should expect to feel clumsy, but practice will help you to develop the skills and adapt models of reflection to suit your own particular needs.

In terms of clinical reasoning that leads to decision making, reflection can be invaluable, not only in developing your own practice but also in learning from other people's perspectives and knowledge. You may need, at times, to reflect alone but it is also possible to reflect with your peers, your mentor or within a group of other nurses.

There are many different frameworks that are available to use when reflecting and no single framework is advocated. What is important is the process of reflection itself and that you choose a framework that you are able to work with. The further reading section pertaining to reflection can be found at the end of this chapter.

What?	While working on a medical ward I was asked to look after an elderly gentleman who had severe respiratory disease. Some of the care assistants said good luck and were complaining about this gentleman, stating he was too lazy to wash himself and it was such a shame that his wife had to do everything at home for him as she was frail. I felt a little upset and shocked by this description of the patient in such a negative way. I decided to assess the patient before I started helping him with his hygiene needs. My assessment showed that he was quite breathless when talking and his respiratory rate was 36 per minute, breathing shallow but regular. I asked him if he would like me to help him to have a wash. He agreed to this but stated he wasn't able to do much because of his breathing. I helped the patient to have a wash in the chair. He managed to wash his face but noticed that even this amount of effort was causing an increase in his breathlessness. So I asked the patient if he would like me to wash the rest of him and he said yes, seeming very relieved and saying I was very kind as on previous days he had been left to manage as best he could with a bowl beside the bed
So what?	This situation had a lot of implications for myself, the ward team and for the patient: • I need to do something about how the care assistants had treated this gentleman. If I don't, I will continue to feel bad and concerned for the patient. • I am junior. I need to talk to my mentor as it is impacting on his care • Need reassurance that I have acted correctly. I think I have. We recently had a lecture about breathlessness and, while I recognize we need to try and encourage as much independence and mobility as possible, I know that breathlessness increases on exertion • I need to find out more about breathing problems and how to nurse patients
Now what?	• Do a literature search to get more information to improve my practice • Spoke to my mentor and she was supportive. This will help me to speak up in the future • She is going to do teaching sessions with the care assistants about breathlessness • My mentor is going to refer the patient to the social worker • I feel positive about the outcome. I am a bit more confident about my own skills • Hadn't thought about referral to a social worker for help. I learned how to do a referral to social services

Table 2.5 What, so what and now what?

It is also useful to consider the following questions in order to help you identify how you access opportunities for reflection and how you might be able to enhance your reflective activities.

Exercise 2.9

Which opportunities do you access for reflection?

? Alone?

? With your mentor?

? Within a group?

? How might you work towards utilizing further opportunities for reflection, and how might these benefit your practice?

? Do you need help and support to develop reflective skills, and how might these benefit your practice?

You may have thought of the following:

- set aside specific time for reflection within the working day or at home
- explore the benefits of lone versus group reflection
- enable you to identify how you feel about situations you encounter
- identify your learning needs
- support the development of evidence-based practice
- help to ensure the delivery of expert nursing for those you provide care for
- talk to others about their experience of reflection
- organize peer support to facilitate reflection
- talk to your mentor to access help with this
- explore different models of reflection to see which model best suits your needs
- ask your personal tutor to help you to develop your reflective skills and guide you in how these might be developed.

Conclusion

This chapter has concentrated on the problems of defining nursing, encouraging you to develop your own understanding of what nursing is, exploring levels of practice achievement and decision making, and using reflection to assist in the process of your development within nursing.

References

Bondy, K. N. (1983) Criterion-referenced definitions for rating scales in clinical evaluation, *Journal of Nursing Education*, 22(9): 376–82.

Burns, S. and Bulman, C. (eds) (2000) *Reflective Practice in Nursing: The Growth of the Professional Practitioner*, 2nd edn., Chapter 2. Oxford: Blackwell Science.

Canadian Association of Midwives (2009) *Midwifery Practice – What is a Midwife?* Available online at www.canadianmidwives.org/midwife.htm (accessed 21 August 2009).

Candela, L., Dalley, K. and Benzel-Lindley, J. (2006) A case for learning-centred curricula, *Journal of Nursing Education*, 45(2): 59–66.

Clements, A. (2007) Know yourself, know your patients, *Nursing Standard*, 22(9): 64.

Concise Oxford Dictionary (1988) 2nd edn. Oxford: Oxford University Press.

Driscoll, J. (1994) Reflective practice for practise – a framework of structured reflection for clinical areas, *Senior Nurse*, 14(1): 47–50.

Henderson, V. (1960) *Basic Principles of Nursing Care*. London: ICN.

Jepson, R. (2007) *Cranberries for Preventing Urinary Tract Infections*. Oxford: The Cochrane Collaboration.

Murphy, J. (2004) Using focused reflection and articulation to promote clinical reasoning: an evidence-based teaching strategy, *National League for Nursing Inc.*, 25(5): 236–41.

Nicholl, H. and Higgins, A. (2004) Reflection in pre-registration curricula, *Journal of Advanced Nursing*, 46(6): 578–85.

Parsons, A. and White, J. (2007) Learning from reflection on intramuscular injections, *Nursing Standard*, 22(17): 35–40.

Reid, B. (1993) 'But we're doing it already': Exploring a response to the concept of reflective practice in order to promote its facilitation, *Nurse Education Today*, 13(4): 305–9.

Royal College of Nursing (RCN) (2000) *Defining Nursing*. London: RCN.

Schön, D. (1983) *The Reflective Practitioner*. New York: Basic Books.

Williamson, G.R., Jenkinson, T. and Proctor-Childs, T. (2008) *Nursing in Contemporary Practice*. Exeter: Learning Matters Ltd.

Further reading

American Nurses Association (ANA) (1980) *Nursing: A Social Policy Statement*. Kansas City, MD: ANA.

Clark, J. (1997) The unique function of the nurse (inaugural Henderson memorial lecture), *International Nursing Review*, 44(5): 144–52.

Cooney, A. (1999) Reflection demystified! Answering some common questions, *British Journal of Nursing*, 8(2): 1530–4.

Gibbs, G. (1988) *Learning by Doing: A Guide to Teaching and Learning Methods*. Oxford: Further Education Unit, Oxford Polytechnic.

International Council of Nurses (ICN) (2002) *The ICN Definition of Nursing*. Geneva: ICN.

Jasper, M. (2003) *Beginning Reflective Practice*. Cheltenham: Nelson Thornes.

Johns, C. (2004) *Becoming a Reflective Practitioner*, 2nd edn. Oxford: Blackwell Publishing.

Keeling, M. (2002) Is midwifery an art? *Journal of Midwifery and Women's Health*, 472: back page editorial.

Kolb, D. (1984) *Experiential Learning: Experience as a Source of Learning and Development*. Upper Saddle River, NJ: Prentice Hall.

Nightingale, F. (1859) *Notes on Nursing: What it Is and What it is Not*. London: Harrison.

Scottish Office Home and Health Department (1991) *The Role and Function of the Professional Nurse*. Edinburgh: Scottish Office Home and Health Department.

Taylor, B.J. (2006) *Reflective Practice: A Guide for Nurses and Midwives*, 2nd edn. Maidenhead: Open University Press.

3 Using evidence-based practice to support decision making

- **Introduction**
- **What does evidence-based practice mean for nurses?**
- **Levels of evidence**
- **Accountability and evidence**
- **Portfolios**
- **How a portfolio can assist reflection, develop clinical reasoning and decision making**
- **Suggestion for completing a portfolio entry**
- **How evidence might affect reasoning processes and the decisions made**
- **Appraising evidence**
- **Critical thinking skills**
- **Conclusion**
- **References**
- **Further reading**

Introduction

Chapter 2 saw the introduction of professional evidence and reflection as important components of decision making. In this chapter, consideration will be given to evidence-based practice and clinical evidence to further support decision making and explore how these influence and impact on decision making. The Nursing and Midwifery Council (NMC) (2008a: 7) now requires nurses to use evidence-based practice as shown in the following quote from the Code: 'You must deliver care based on the best available evidence or best practice' and 'You must ensure any advice you give is evidence based …'.

You may be wondering why evidence-based practice has assumed such a high profile in nursing during the past decade. Again, the drive to enable nursing to become a true profession has had a large part to play in this. As part of this drive, research in nursing has gathered speed and volume. In addition, changes in society, the complexities of health care, patient choice and assertiveness have demanded that nurses are able to validate their care and to explain reasons for care decisions. It is obviously impossible to explain ourselves if we are not up to date in our spheres of work. Gone are the days when a nurse could qualify, be placed on the register and remain there without any further study/updating. In fact, there are specific requirements by our professional bodies with regard to the minimum of updating that must occur in order to continue to remain on the live register (NMC, 2008b).

What does evidence-based practice mean for nurses?

Evidence-based practice, as far as nursing was concerned, grew out of all of the above. However, some consideration needs to be given as to what evidence-based practice and clinical evidence actually mean for nurses. There has been much discussion in the nursing literature about this; it is interesting however, to look at an earlier piece of work (albeit from the medical sphere) that did in fact 'set the scene' so to speak.

Sackett et al. (1996: 71) offered the following definition: 'Evidence Based Medicine is the conscientious, explicit and judicious use of current best evidence in making decisions about the care of individual patients.'

It was interesting in this discourse that the concepts of clinical expertise, patient choice and values must accompany the use of evidence to make decisions. This sentiment has also been expressed in the nursing literature (Kitson, 2002; Dale, 2005). There is a need to consider what constitutes evidence as far as nursing is concerned. Some clues to this will have been observed from the 'add on framework' in Chapter 1 and the concept of reflection in Chapter 2.

Levels of evidence

Evidence for making/explaining/justifying decisions comes from a variety of sources. It is important to remember that each type of evidence has advantages and disadvantages. Therefore, in setting out levels of evidence, you have to consider the advantages and disadvantages of the evidence in the context of the type of patient/client group you are caring for. The other factor that will affect your decision making is the proliferation of information now available from a variety of sources such as the Internet, health care journals and textbooks. It is obviously impossible to read thoroughly such a large amount of material. Interestingly, this has been identified in the medical literature where Grol and Grimshaw (2003) have written of (medical) clinicians' difficulties in keeping apace with the advances in health care knowledge. This problem is equally applicable to nursing. A consideration of levels of evidence can help you to select material that will effectively support decision making.

Exercise 3.1

What do you consider to be the main sources of evidence in nursing?

You may have considered the following:

- research (quantitative and qualitative)
- literature reviews
- audit
- journals
- databases and the Internet
- expert clinical opinion
- policies and guidelines
- textbooks.

We now go through each type of evidence in turn.

Research

Research is often placed at the top of the list, particularly randomized controlled trials (RCTs) that are considered in some quarters to be the 'gold standard' for evidence. (Sackett et al., 1996; Jennings and Loan, 2001). RCTs and also systematic reviews of research literature may help to evaluate nursing interventions. RCTs are studies in which individuals are allocated randomly to receive an intervention and then the individuals are followed up to see if the interventions have had an effect. The results are then compared to individuals who have not received the intervention in order to determine whether the intervention itself has made a difference. Systematic reviews of studies compare the results of a variety of research studies on the same topic. These can then be evaluated to see whether studies that are of good quality can be combined to demonstrate they produce similar results, thereby lending reliability to the research findings if similar results are found.

However, when it comes to the consideration of the patient's experience, attitudes and beliefs, the required evidence requires a different approach from quantitative research to obtain appropriate evidence. Qualitative research tends to be used to gain insight into people's attitudes, behaviours, value systems, concerns, motivations and cultural lifestyles. Qualitative research does not tend to focus on statistical forms of analysis (Mason, 1996) and therefore is seen by some researchers as less rigorous than quantitative research. However, statistical (quantitative) studies often do not produce richness of data required to illuminate the themes that emerge from qualitative studies. Hence, the validity of research methods used will be dependent on the topic and aspects addressed, and what the researcher wants to explore.

Literature reviews

A literature review can often help provide an objective view of available evidence. The purpose of a literature review is to gather information about a particular topic from many different but relevant sources (Timmins and McCabe, 2005). Literature reviews are often undertaken in relation to specific spheres of a nursing speciality or topic.

Many journals that publish literature reviews may well be international, which can prove to be a useful global view on a topic, but it is important to remember that what may be acceptable in one country may not be so in another.

Audit

Audit and feedback may also prove a useful source of evidence. Audit in the context relating to health care means a review process to check that existing standards of care are being met. For example, an infection control audit might involve an observer measuring how often staff in the practice area wash their hands while undertaking care. Feedback from audit can indicate whether standards of care in relation to hand hygiene are maintained. From these findings it can be communicated whether any changes are needed or current practice continues. This may serve as a useful evidence base especially where quality of care is concerned. Audit can also be repeated at a later date to ascertain if there has been an improvement from the previous performance in the light of any changes made.

Journals

A wealth of journals both national and international now exist within nursing and midwifery literature. They have the advantage, particularly over textbooks, of being more up to date as they are published on a regular basis and within a shorter timespan. Nurses do need to take care in selecting journal material: some journal articles are subject to peer review, others are not. This needs to be borne in mind when selecting evidence to support practice decisions. Peer review is the process of asking people who are considered experts in a particular field to critically appraise the article that has been submitted for publication. Peer reviewing journal articles helps to make the material more credible by seeking such a review from experts.

Databases and the Internet

Bibliographic databases (Medline, Cinahl, Embase) are useful for general searches and Internet sources now play a greater part in providing evidence. However, some Internet sources are not credible and care needs to be taken when using such a source. The material on some Internet sites is likely to be generalized and not subject to expert input and review. Good sources of Internet evidence use acknowledged experts to source their material, for example, government databases such as the Department of Health (DoH) website.

Expert clinical opinion

The importance of expert clinical opinion must not be overlooked. For example, experts in a particular field may not have the required research-based evidence to support a particular intervention. However, they may have observed that a specific intervention works in a given situation. Ideally, research would follow on from this observation but this may not always be the case. However, expert opinion should not be discounted when considering evidence.

Policies and guidelines

Policies, guidelines and formularies are all credible sources of evidence and, provided they are updated regularly, they are reliable. The sources of policies and guidelines could be local or national. For example, a national policy may be produced by the National Patient Safety Agency (NPSA) as is the case in relation to guidance on blood transfusion care delivery. Local policies and guidelines may be produced by an organization to reflect the local situation. For example, there are a variety of machines that can measure a person's blood glucose. The policy and guideline produced, in conjunction with the care associated with this equipment, would reflect the specific meter in use.

Textbooks

Textbooks are useful for material that is not subject to change over a prolonged period. For example, a textbook on the topic of physiology is likely to be relevant for a reasonably long period. However, textbooks may be updated by publishing a new addition with the latest material included. It is important when using a textbook to ensure the latest edition is utilized.

When considering best available evidence, the evidence may not always be conclusive. Try Exercise 3.2. to compare evidence from a variety of sources.

Exercise 3.2

There is a belief that cranberry juice can help to prevent urinary tract infections. Try searching for some evidence on this and then classify the evidence into the different categories. Enquire in one of your placements what the general opinion about this is. What does a specialist have to say about this matter?

You may wish to include this exercise in your portfolio – a topic that is addressed shortly.

Accountability and evidence

In Chapter 1 a brief reference was made to the topic of accountability and to whom the qualified nurse is accountable. Accountability requires that a nurse will be called upon to explain the rationale for decisions made, or not made, as the case may be. The ultimate arena for such an explanation would be a court of law or a coroner's inquiry but there are other occasions when this may be required, for example, as the result of a complaint from a patient or other person. It is clear that our reasoning and decision making must be based on sound evidence and knowledge. Therefore, the nurse must select appropriate, effective and up-to-date evidence to justify reasoning and decision making.

Portfolios

Another source of evidence that can be particularly useful in your decision making is the compilation of a portfolio. A portfolio in this sense has been defined as: 'A collection of evidence, usually in written form, of both the products and processes of learning. It attests to achievements of both personal and professional development, by providing a critical analysis of its contents' (McMullan et al., 2003: 289).

As a student on a pre-registration course, you will be required to compile a portfolio of evidence to support your learning. Your portfolio may be partly or wholly assessed by your higher education institution but there are common elements present in all portfolios. Portfolios will also consist of private matter that you may not wish to divulge to other parties, and information to be shared with others such as mentors or personal tutors. Specific guidance as to content will also be specified by your higher education institution but, generally speaking, the following is a list of what might be included:

- reflective accounts from clinical practice
- what you have actually learned from your clinical practice
- reports from insight and other relevant visits to, say, specialist facilities (these are sometimes called witness statements)
- analyses of critical incidents
- annotated bibliographies to support clinical practice
- feedback, advice, comments from mentors in clinical practice
- work products; that is, care plans.

Note: This is not an exhaustive list.

The literature surrounding portfolios reports variable reactions. McMullan's (2008) study from the nursing literature has identified that while they are considered to be good for providing a collection of evidence for clinical learning and awareness of students' strengths and weaknesses, some respondents in this study felt that there was too much emphasis on assessment and academic skill and insufficiently integrated theory and practice. However, an American study that polled respondents from more general backgrounds (Brown, 2002) highlights advantages particularly related to learning through work and mentors.

How a portfolio can assist reflection, develop clinical reasoning and decision making

In considering how a portfolio can assist with reflection, clinical reasoning and decision making, examine the following specimen portfolio entry.

This following portfolio extract highlights the importance of liaising with physiotherapists to help mobilize patients safely; this knowledge can then be incorporated into plans for care and ensure that co-workers follow such plans.

During a placement where waiting list patients underwent orthopaedic surgery, I spent a period of time with a senior physiotherapist who was advising patients who had undergone total hip replacements. One aspect of this was related to the importance of undertaking muscle strengthening exercises in order to provide stability and successful movement post-operatively.

I felt that this was an aspect of care for which I had previously received little input and on discussing with the physiotherapist, the importance was stressed to me that patients do need to receive reminders and supervision from nurses in order to provide continuity of care and a successful outcome for this procedure. As the physiotherapist said, they are severely stretched for time and the number of patients that they can see, so it is vital that nurses appropriately encourage and supervise patients to undertake their specified exercises. I decided to investigate the background to this element further and include it in my profile.

From the sample portfolio entry, the following was identified as having been learned by the student:

- muscle function
- rectification of prior muscle weakness
- regaining of normal posture and mobility
- maintenance of effective circulation
- prevention of deep vein thrombosis (DVT) formation
- the importance of effective pain relief in order to carry out exercises.

Exercise 3.3

How will this portfolio exercise aid clinical reasoning and decision making in future clinical practice?

Considering what was learned from this situation and reflecting on how this knowledge will be applied in future clinical practice needs to be specified in the portfolio entry. As a follow-up (at a later point) other elements may be added. Some points to consider might be:

- How many patients undergoing total hip replacement are at risk of DVT?

- If a patient does develop DVT, what are the implications for that patient?

- What are the resource implications that may result from this?

Note: You may have noticed that the follow-up points suggested would probably be addressed at a later point in the course such as at Stage 3 of the 'add on framework'.

Suggestion for completing a portfolio entry

Your portfolio entries should relate to your stage on the 'add on framework' for decision making. How you complete your portfolio is up to you. However, it is absolutely vital that however you develop your portfolio, you need to identify what you have learned from the examples you include and, if possible, how this learning will impact on your current and future practice. It is important to remember that practitioners draw on multiple sources of knowledge in their practice (Rycroft-Malone et al., 2004). You may include published evidence along with your portfolio entries but do remember to read such evidence thoroughly so that you can explain how it relates to practice and, in particular, decision making.

Examples of how portfolio entries may be built up at various stages in the course are outlined below.

Portfolio entry: Stage I

This stage should reflect on your experiences and part of your reflection might be to consider how and why the decision was made.

> I was working on my first placement and was asked to take a patient's daily vital signs of temperature, pulse and respirations. The patient's temperature had risen from 37 to 38. I decided I had better let my mentor know this as it seemed a bit high.
>
> My mentor asked me to increase the frequency of the observations to four-hourly.
>
> I was talking to my mentor later and asked her why she decided that four-hourly observations were necessary. She explained that the patient had a pyrexia

and the routine is that if a patient has a raised temperature, you usually increase the frequency to four-hourly as you need to monitor the patient who might be developing an infection.

I have learned from this that:

❶ the frequency of observations will depend on the baseline observation you make on patients
❷ I need to think about why changes in results occur and not just record them
❸ I need to talk to my mentor further and find out what else might need to be done for a patient who suddenly develops a high temperature.

Portfolio entry: Stage 2

Stage 2 in the 'add on framework' expects you to start looking at peer/expert opinion.

I was helping my mentor to do the medicine round for our group of patients. One patient was taking oral steroids and my mentor said she had been on these for some time so I would need to do a urine test on her to check for glucose in her urine. I didn't have time to ask my mentor why this needed to be done.

I was thinking about this when I got home and looked up prednisolone (this was the steroid the patient was taking) in the British National Formulary. I learned from doing this that:

❶ steroids can cause glycosuria
❷ I know now that I need to check a patient's urine for glycosuria when they are on steroid therapy, particularly if it is prolonged therapy
❸ I also know that I need to report the findings so that everyone knows to check the urine regularly and to ensure that I document this in the patient's records
❹ From reading about record-keeping (NMC, 2009), I know that I must ensure that entries into records are clear, legible, factual, and that as a student I need to get all entries countersigned by a registered nurse.

Portfolio entry: Stage 3

At Stage 3 of the 'add on framework' you need to identify how you can learn from policies, guidelines for care and from research. An entry in your portfolio might be as follows.

As part of my current placement I spent some time with the diabetic nurse specialist. She was very popular with the patients and seemed to know an awful lot about her patients and her subject. I decided to explore whether a nurse specialist in the care of people with long-term conditions actually has a beneficial effect on patients.

I found an article that addresses the issue of effectiveness of nurse case managers in improving health outcomes in three major diseases (Sutherland and Hayter, 2009). The findings of this study support the beneficial effects on patient outcomes. It is therefore worthwhile to include this evidence in my portfolio to support my specialist visit. This article demonstrates that the nature of this type of nursing is effective both clinically and economically. Referrals to such nurse specialists can prevent or reduce complications from long-term conditions such as diabetes and by so doing can improve patient outcomes.

I realize that I need to consider suggesting referrals to nurse specialists when I am caring for and managing a group of patients.

I will also try to ensure that I can spend time with the relevant nurse specialists in future placements, and will read about their roles before I visit them so that I can discuss their role in a more informed way.

Exercise 3.4

For a possible entry in your own portfolio, reflect on the importance of a particular intervention in your own area. (Seek different types of evidence to support your account.)

Portfolio evidence from even a short clinical experience can have widespread applications elsewhere. This is the value of reviewing and reflecting on your clinical experience. It is also the ideal opportunity when you meet with your mentors to jointly discuss such examples of evidence. As you progress through your pre-registration course you will refine your portfolio, often as a result of feedback from your tutors and mentors and further clinical experience. Your evidence will become increasingly complex and detailed (again refer back to the 'add on framework' that was introduced in Chapter 1).

How evidence might affect reasoning processes and the decisions made

The following situation can illustrate how evidence may affect your reasoning and decision making.

Exercise 3.5   Clostridium difficile infections

There is a great deal of concern about clostridium difficile infections. The result-
ant diarrhoea is distressing for patients and, in some cases, life-threatening. You
will know of the emphasis on hygiene issues in connection with this infective
process. You may also be aware of the role that some antibiotics play in relation to
the development of diarrhoea. You might have become aware of the role that
probiotics play in the possible prevention of antibiotic-induced diarrhoea including clostridium difficile. A broad-based literature search taking in a number of
disciplines may well yield a good proportion of evidence that can help to justify
the decision to provide probiotic drinks to vulnerable patients.

❶ Look up some literature on the use of probiotics in clostridium difficile.
❷ Does the evidence that you can find support the above?

Evidence may well change previous ideas on topics. However, given the amount of
evidence available, especially when evidence relates to a number of disciplines, it can
make reviewing the literature an enormous task.

Having looked at a Cochrane review of probiotics in connection with clostridium
difficile (Pillai and Nelson, 2009), the review of the literature relating to this finds that
the use of probiotics in clostridium difficile is not warranted. Reviews such as this are
really useful as they have appraised a great deal of literature on your behalf. This not
only saves you time, but Cochrane reviews are undertaken by experts in the relevant
field. The Cochrane database is a very good example of an Internet-based service that
gives you efficient access to reliable sources of evidence, reviewed from a number of
perspectives.

Appraising evidence

If you review the 'add on framework' in Chapter 1, you will see that as you progress
through your pre-registration courses and beyond, your evidence will of necessity
become more complex. You will become aware of wider sources of evidence and
eventually you will begin to appraise more research-based work to support clinical
reasoning and decision making. In order to do this, you will need to be able to appraise
the effectiveness, reliability and validity of such work.

Reliability is the extent to which data collection methods will collect the same data
on repeated occasions, and validity is the extent to which the research measures what it
intends to measure (Lindsay, 2007).

Pre-registration courses do include material on how to appraise research but it is a
task that takes much time and effort. For instance, in appraising a quantitative piece of
research, you will often need to assess whether the right statistical test has been used.

How would you know? Unless you have an in-depth knowledge of statistics, it is unlikely that you will be able to make a safe decision about this. In selecting quantitative research, therefore, you will need to be very careful about using such evidence. How then might you look to increasing the complexity of evidence without encountering problems of reliability and validity?

You might make use of specialists who will have experience in selecting and utilizing complex evidence. You might make use of experienced nurses within your placement or, if you visit specialist clinics/departments, these may well be run by specialist nurses and they are, by reason of their job remit, a source of reliable information. In addition, they will be using sound evidence for their clinical practice role.

Also, participation in multiprofessional teamwork will often identify sources of evidence that you perhaps had not realized existed, evidence that is undertaken from a perspective other than nursing. This can expand your understanding of care that is given to patients as you get a fuller picture of evidence that could pertain to the patient's problem.

Exercise 3.6   Ward observation

In an appropriate setting and at an appropriate time in your course, enquire if you may observe a ward medical round/case conference. These are often learning opportunities, especially if junior doctors or medical students are involved. Make a point of following up elements that you did not understand. It will be useful to try and gather some evidence for your portfolio as this will often identify up-to-date and relevant evidence for your practice. *Note*: You need to be fairly well advanced in your pre-registration course to gain advantage from this exercise.

Critical thinking skills

Critical thinking is a mental process of evaluating information, reflecting on the meaning and examining the offered evidence and, in reviewing evidence, you will start to develop critical thinking skills. The next step in critical thinking is to use reasoning to start to form judgements about the information you have been exposed to (Marquis and Huston, 2009). As a student you need to develop critical thinking, not only within your theoretical assignments, but during the course of your practice experience and development of your portfolio.. The written assignments you undertake as part of the programme that you are undertaking are invaluable in helping you develop as a critical thinker. It is also useful to use your portfolio material to develop your critical thinking skills. If you have read a research-based article relating to some aspect of care you have been involved in, you need to identify why and how the research is relevant to your client group, compare the findings with what you have experienced and already know, make a judgement about how these findings could/would influence your practice in the future, and reflect on how you will incorporate this new information into your future practice. Hence, critical thinking involves an element of reflection.

Critical thinking is different to problem-solving and decision making in that problem-solving relates to analysing a difficult situation and is a step within the process of decision making. Critical thinking is a broader concept that requires you to examine and form a judgement about the relevance of information or systems to the patient/ client group that you are caring for, and the context in which the caring takes place.

Sound evidence-based care is a requirement in achieving Stage 3 in the decision-making framework and for achieving Bondy Level 4 in relation to practice. Reading and using evidence is not enough. You need to develop the ability to read, evaluate, review and provide sound rationales for why you would use a specific piece of evidence to support the decisions you make about the way care is delivered to a patient or group of patients. Critical thinking skills are necessary for this and will help you to justify your actions should you be held to account for decisions made in specific situations. Put simply, critical thinking means going beyond obvious findings to make informed, purposeful judgements and, to think critically, one must first have a knowledge base on which to reason (Fowler, 1998).

Consider the following example in Exercise 3.7 that could be applicable within any branch of nursing/midwifery.

Exercise 3.7

A patient you are caring for has an open wound on their lower calf. You are asked to renew this dressing. A dry dressing is requested in the patient's plan of care. You remove the dressing with some difficulty as it has adhered to the wound.

❶ Is this the best choice of wound dressing for this type of wound?
❷ How would you decide on which dressing might be appropriate?
❸ What evidence would you base your decision on?

Clinical experience is necessary for the development of critical reasoning and decision-making skills (Toofany, 2008), with a knowledge base in wound care being necessary in order for you to reason through a sound approach to this patient's wound care.

You may have thought of the following:

❶ You recognize the importance of assessment as a prerequisite for good wound care (Gould, 1984). You are aware that scientific evidence has led to a change from dry to moist wound healing management (Bolton et al., 1990; Lait and Smith, 1998). The ideal wound dressing is one that provides a moist environment, is comfortable for the patient, removes necrotic material, promotes the production of granulation tissue, stimulates re-epthelialization and is cost-effective (Griffith, 1991) as well as reducing pain and tenderness for the patient (Lait and Smith, 1998).

❷ You recognize the need to protect the wound from drying and trauma on removal of the dressing (Lait and Smith, 1998). You are also aware that there are many dressings and therefore need to balance efficient and effective wound care against cost-effectiveness (Lazarus et al., 1994; Griffiths Jones, 1991). The variety of wound care products can be confusing for nurses. You may refer to the local wound care formulary produced by specialists in wound care that can help you in selecting the correct product for this patient.

❸ The evidence you have based your decision on will be scientific research, local expert opinion and your knowledge regarding the literature available regarding wounds and wound care products, as well as your assessment of this individual client.

Conclusion

In conclusion, it is necessary that you select evidence that comes from a credible source and will expand your knowledge. Following the 'add on framework' will help you do this. You cannot expect to utilize complex evidence early on in your clinical experience. You need experience in practice first, and then you can build on this by exploring which evidence is effective in supporting your care delivery and the decisions you make. Ineffective evidence is unsafe and decisions made without relevant evidence may put patients/clients at risk of harm.

As a student, the most immediate source of help for assessing evidence are your mentors. In addition, it may be helpful to discuss evidence you have read with your peers and your personal tutor.

References

Bolton, L., Pirone, L., Chew, J. and Lydon, M. (1990) Dressing effects on wound healing, *Wounds*, 2(4): 126–34.

Brown, J.O. (2002) Know thyself: the impact of portfolio development on adult learning, *Adult Education Quarterly*, 52(3): 228–45.

Dale, A.E. (2005) Evidence based practice: compatability with nursing, *Nursing Standard* 19(40): 48–53.

Fowler, L.P. (1998) Improving critical thinking in nursing practice, *Journal for Nurses in Staff Development*, 14(4): 183–7.

Gould, D. (1984) Clinical Forum, *Nursing Mirror*, 159(16): 3–6.

Griffiths, G. (1991) Choosing a dressing, *Nursing Times*, 87(36): 84–90.

Griffiths-Jones, A. (1991) Wound care: can the nursing process help? *Professional Nurse*, January: 208–12.

Grol, R. and Grimshaw, J. (2003) From best evidence to best practice: effective implementation of change in patients' care, *The Lancet*, 362(9391): 1225–30.

Jennings, B.M and Loan, L.A. (2001) Misconceptions among nurses about evidence based practice, *Journal of Nursing Scholarship*, 33(2): 121–7.

Kitson, A. (2002) Recognising relationships: reflections on evidence based practice, *Nursing Inquiry*, 9(3): 179–86.

Lait, M. and Smith, L. (1998) Wound management: a literature review, *Journal of Clinical Nursing*, 7: 11–17.

Lazarus, G., Cooper, D., Knighton, D., Margolis, D., Pecaroro, R., Rodeheaver, G. and Robinson, M. (1994) Definitions and guidelines for the assessment of wounds and evaluation of healing, *Archives of Dermatology*, 130: 487–93.

Lindsay, B. (2007) *Understanding Research and Eevidence-based Practice.* Exeter: Reflect Press.

Marquis, B.L. and Huston, C.J. (2009) *Leadership Roles and Management Functions*, 6th edn. London: Wolters Kluwer Health/Lippincott, Williams & Wilkins.

Mason, J. (1996) *Qualitative Researching*, 1st edn. London: Sage Publications.

McMullan, M. (2008) Using portfolios for clinical practice learning and assessment: the pre-registration student's perception, *Nurse Education Today*, 28(7): 873–9.

McMullan, M., Endacott, R., Gray, M.A., Jasper, M., Miller, C.M.L., Scholes, J. and Webb, C. (2003) Portfolios and assessment of competence: a review of the literature, *Journal of Advanced Nursing*, 41(3): 283–94.

Nursing and Midwifery Council (NMC) (2008a) *The Code: Standards of Conduct, Performance and Ethics for Nurses and Midwives.* London: NMC.

Nursing and Midwifery Council (NMC) (2008b) *The Prep Handbook.* London: NMC.

Nursing and Midwifery Council (NMC) (2009) *Record Keeping: Guidance for Nurses and Midwives.* London: NMC.

Pillai, A. and Nelson, R.L. (2009) Probiotics for treatment of clostridium difficile-associated colitis in adults (Review), *Cochrane Database of Systematic Reviews*, 23(1): CD 004611.

Rycroft-Malone, J., Seers, K., Titchen, A., Harvey, G., Kitson, A. and McCormack, B. (2004) What counts as evidence based practice? *Journal of Advanced Nursing*, 47(1): 81–90.

Sackett, D.L., Rosenberg, W.M.C., Muir Gray, J.A., Haynes, R.B. and Richardson, W.S. (1996) Evidence based medicine: what it is and what it isn't, *British Medical Journal*, 312(7023): 71–2.

Sutherland, D. and Hayter, M. (2009) Structures review: evaluating the effectiveness of nurse case managers in improving health outcomes in three major chronic diseases, *Journal of Clinical Nursing*, 18(21): 2978–92.

Timmins, F. and McCabe, C. (2005) How to conduct an effective literature search, *Nursing Standard*, 20(11): 41–7.

Toofany, S. (2008) Critical thinking among nurses, *Nursing Management*, 19(4): 28–31.

Further reading

Evidence-based Nursing, London: BMJ Publishing Group Ltd (a publication that reviews evidence from a wide variety of scholarly health care journals).

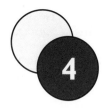

Getting the most out of your mentor when making decisions

4

Introduction

We have explored what nursing is and the need for evidence to support nursing practice. In this chapter, we need to explore the role of the mentor with regard to helping us to learn from experience. During your education programme, your mentor is a key person in helping you to transfer the knowledge and skills that you have acquired into real-life situations. Spouse (2001) refers to this as transferring knowledge in waiting to knowledge in use. The decisions that you make regarding patients using your skills and knowledge should be a key element in terms of bridging the perceived theory-to-practice divide. In applying your skills and theoretical knowledge, you will be able to make the most appropriate decisions with your patient regarding their clinical care. This chapter focuses on how to get the most out of your mentor in relation to this transition.

A little about mentorship

Mentorship roles and responsibilities were redefined by the Nursing and Midwifery Council (NMC) in 2006 (NMC, 2008), with mentors having to demonstrate competence in the following domains:

- establishing effective working relationships
- facilitation of learning
- assessment and accountability
- evaluation of learning
- creating an environment for learning
- context of practice
- evidence-based practice
- leadership.

As you can identify from the domains the mentor has to demonstrate competence in, the mentor's role is less that of an educator and more the role of facilitator, supporter and evaluator of learning. This does not mean that the mentor will not teach students but the emphasis is on the role of facilitator and role model, who has the knowledge and expertise to provide appropriate learning opportunities for students. This role then culminates in evaluating the student's learning and making a judgement as to the level of competence achieved by the student.

What will your mentor mean to you?

Your mentor is the key person in facilitating, assessing and evaluating your learning in your practice placement. The mentor is also the expert in knowing which experiences and opportunities are available for you to access. Their role is to help match those experiences with the goals that either you or a previous mentor has identified as important for you to work on. In addition, the mentor may need to help you to adjust those goals to assist you in developing realistic expectations from the placement.

In demonstrating competence in the domains of mentorship, the mentor should fulfil the four main activities that have been ascribed to mentoring:

1. supervision
2. teaching while engaged in expert practice activities
3. assessment feedback
4. emotional support to students in their care.

Source: Philips et al. (1996); Spouse (1996).

We now go through each of these in turn:

Supervision

From the first placement you experience, your mentor will be observing your performance and making sure that the care you deliver is correctly undertaken and appropriate for that particular patient. They will also prompt you and make suggestions as you go along. Your mentor is accountable for what you do. This means that supervision will involve a lot of scrutiny of you initially but, as you progress along your course, the supervision will become less direct as your clinical expertise, knowledge and decision-making abilities increase as a result of prior learning.

Teaching while engaged in expert practice activities

Your mentor will be able to talk you through activities that you are learning, and will explain why the care that you deliver is adapted in a particular way with a specific patient. Your teaching in the university will introduce you to principles of care and how to deliver care and undertake skills in a specific way. The mentor's role is to help you to transfer your learning, and understand how certain activities undertaken with patients may be adapted to suit the specific needs of a particular person, while still being a safe approach to care.

Assessment feedback

You are a learner within a placement area and will need feedback on your performance. Much of this feedback will be informal feedback from your mentor. This may be verbal or may be written feedback depending on the situation and whether an action plan may be required for your further development. However, the purpose of the mentor is also to give formal feedback to the student through assessing your abilities against the criteria required from you at a specific point in your course. This means that the mentor will have to make a formal judgement about your development, giving you advice about how you can develop your performance in the future. If the formal feedback is positive, this can give you a tremendous boost to your morale and can help you to identify how much you have learned within a placement, and how this can be built on in the future.

Constructive feedback may make you feel as though you have not achieved as much as you would have liked. However, the mentor's role is to be honest and help you to identify exactly what you need to do in the future in order to improve your performance. This feedback can help to increase your self-awareness and, if you approach it in a positive manner, can be a valuable and productive learning experience.

Emotional support to students in their care

Nursing is not only a physically demanding profession, but can also be emotionally demanding at times. Remember, your mentor was a student just like you. If you feel overwhelmed in the placement, or are having difficulties because you are upset about a person's difficult circumstances, you can talk about this to your mentor. They will share their own experiences with you and are aware of the resources available to you to help you cope in these situations. Nurses have to cope with situations that most of the public never have to face and it does not mean you are a failure if you ask for help and advice with your feelings.

You may also be having a difficult time outside of the placement environment. These, for example, may be financial difficulties, family or relationship problems. If you have problems like this that may affect your performance in placement, do let your mentor know. They will not be able to solve these problems for you, but they will be aware of sources of support that you can access. In keeping your mentor informed, it can help to explain why your performance may be affected at times, and can prevent your mentor attributing your performance to lack of interest or enthusiasm.

Maximizing time with your mentor

As a student it is important that you maximize your time with your mentor as they have many demands on their time apart from their teaching role. The pressure of clinical commitments and lack of available time can create an increase of pressure on individual nurses (Clarke et al., 2003; Davies et al., 1999; Neary, 1997). So it is important that as a student you maximize the learning opportunities you have with your mentor and start to think about how you can get the most from your mentor. Thinking about the strategies you can use will help in reducing pressure on your mentor while at the same time learning from their expertise.

Exercise 4.1

Reflect on the experiences you have had with your mentor. Remember to use a model of reflection to do this. Driscoll's (1994) model is extremely useful: what, so what, now what?

From your reflection identify:

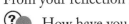 How have you maximized your learning from your mentor?

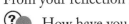 How have your mentors helped you to understand the decisions you/they have made about nursing care?

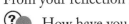 How will you maximize your mentor's role in developing your decision making abilities in the future?

Review your portfolio evidence to help you to do this. It will also help to reflect on the 'add on framework' of decision making when you undertake this exercise.

Reflecting back on your experiences with your mentor not only can help to identify what you have learned, but can also help you to identify an action plan to increase your learning in the future. It may be that, on reflection, you realize that you will need to develop your questioning skills to increase your understanding of your mentor's decision making processes. Alternatively, it can help you to identify how much your decision making processes have improved as a result of your learning in your placement.

Exercise 4.2

Review the goals you have developed for your current placement.

 What influenced you in developing these goals?

 On reflection, are these goals realistic?

 If not, why not?

 If they are, why are they?

 How do your goals for the placement relate to the development of your decision making abilities?

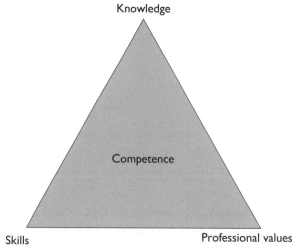 Do you need to adjust your goals to reflect a decision making approach?

Developing competence

In working towards becoming a registered nurse or midwife, you need to develop your competence as a practitioner. Developing competence necessitates working at the knowledge, skills and professional values that you have and demonstrate.

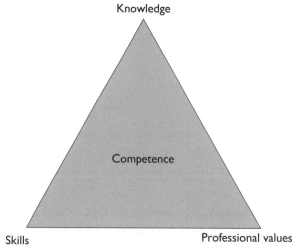

Figure 4.1 Elements of competence

These three elements are important components that the mentor assesses before they can make a judgement in relation to your competence.

Competence

In order to become a registered practitioner, the student has to demonstrate that they can undertake nursing activities. This is the skills element of competence. However, this by itself is not enough. The nurse has to use knowledge to underpin actions, and to be able to make an appropriate decision with or for a person.

Knowledge

If the nurse lacks knowledge, they may not be aware of certain things that need to be done, or may deliver inappropriate care, or even cause harm to a person. For example, certain medicines for constipation act as a bulking agent in the bowel, for example, Fybogel. This bulking agent necessitates the person taking them to have a good fluid intake in order to prevent the bulking agent causing a blockage in the bowel and the person becoming more constipated. If this advice is not given to the patient, or the nurse fails to encourage and monitor that the patient is maintaining an adequate fluid intake, this may cause unnecessary harm and discomfort to the patient.

Professional values

Care may be delivered to a person using a sound knowledge base and safe clinical skills but if professional values are not part of this implementation, this can also be detrimental to a person's well-being. Consider the nurse who takes a person's blood pressure. The nurse may technically be very able and get an accurate blood pressure reading. The same nurse may also be able to interpret the results and make appropriate decisions to act in the best interest of the patient's physical health. However, if the nurse has no interaction with the patient, and leaves the patient's body unduly exposed after the procedure, walking away without giving the patient any reassurance or explanation, this may increase the patient's anxiety, make them angry and leave them feeling less of a person and more of an object. This nurse has caused emotional harm to that person, and may even increase their blood pressure if they are angry or anxious following the procedure. If left exposed, they have also failed to protect that person's dignity. The caring, supportive approach of the nurse is as vital as the knowledge and skill element.

On the other hand, you may have a nurse who is very caring but does not have the knowledge and skill necessary to deliver care. This is as unacceptable as the nurse who does not demonstrate appropriate professional values. The effective nurse is the person who is skilled, has a sound knowledge base and demonstrates appropriate professional values. This is the nurse who demonstrates competence and gains the trust and respect of her patients.

Exercise 4.3

Think about each of these elements of nursing care. Identify why each element must be demonstrated before your mentor can make a judgement about your competence.

If you have acquired specific skills but have no underpinning knowledge, you will be able to perform a skill but will not have the ability to judge when that skill might be required for a patient/service user.

If you have lots of theoretical knowledge but cannot perform a skill, the patient/service user will not receive the care required in a given situation.

Acquiring knowledge and skills that have been applied to decide on a plan of action is beneficial in functioning as a nurse but if you do not have the right approach to a client/service user, that is, appropriate professional values, the patient/service user may feel depersonalized and lacking in value as an individual. For example, a patient asks you for a commode. You may have cleaned the commode prior to use, helped the patient to get onto the commode safely and provided them with toilet paper but, if you complain that they do not really need to empty their bowels yet again in the hearing of other patients and their visitors, you have failed to protect their dignity and failed to value them as a vulnerable person who has feelings. When assessing your competence, your mentor will be assessing all three components. Failure to demonstrate all three elements will result in certain competences not being awarded to you as a student.

The decision making ability of the nurse/midwife is not only dependent on acquiring knowledge, skills and professional values, but is also dependent on your application of these things in any given situation. Developing your reasoning and decision making ability necessitates you learning from your mentors how they combine their knowledge, skills and professional values to arrive at a course of action with/for a specific person.

This is why it is important to maximize the benefit of your access to a variety of registered practitioners. When making decisions, there is often no single course of action in most situations (there are, of course, exceptions to this). Individual practitioners may differ in their approach to decision making and this is often reflected in their preferred learning styles.

How learning styles inform learning to reason and making decisions

In addition to role and time pressures, mentors have to readjust every few weeks to new students, all of whom may like to learn in quite different ways. This can pose an additional challenge for mentors.

While it is not the remit of this chapter to explore different learning styles in depth, it is important to consider how you learn best and what you need to work on in order to get the most out of your experiences. It is extremely useful to do this before you go onto a placement so you can discuss this with your mentor at your preliminary interviews.

Exercise 4.4

Think about how you learn most effectively; what makes you want to learn? What hinders your learning?

Learning styles

Nursing involves a range of activities in which we need to apply a range of skills and you will need to utilize a range of learning styles in order to achieve competence. You can also learn to develop specific learning styles (Sharples, 2009) by reflecting and analysing why you made certain decisions in clinical situations. Through reflection and analysis you can begin to identify the learning style you have used, decide if it is appropriate, and begin to think about whether a different learning style might have been more appropriate in any given situation. In addition, your mentor may prefer a different learning style to yours and this could be a potential source of conflict. If your mentor is a pragmatist and likes to get on with things and act quickly when your preferred learning style is that of a reflector, the mentor may misunderstand you. The mentor may think you lack confidence or are reluctant to access new learning opportunities that could affect your relationship with the mentor.

Honey and Mumford (1992) describe four different learning styles:

❶ activists
❷ reflectors
❸ theorists
❹ pragmatists.

Activists

These individuals thrive on the challenge of new experiences but tend to get bored with longer-term implementation and consolidation.

Reflectors

These individuals tend to ponder experiences from a variety of perspectives and tend to be cautious individuals. They like to think things through carefully.

Theorists

These individuals are quite logical individuals who like to assimilate information into sound theories. They tend to be quite analytical.

Pragmatists

These individuals search out new ideas and like to get on with things and act quickly. They like making practical decisions and solving problems.

Exercise 4.5

Look back at what you wrote about how you like to learn. Compare your thoughts with Honey and Mumford's learning styles. Which type of learning style/s do you prefer?

Nursing requires us to make decisions in many different situations. Some situations necessitate a quick response as in an emergency situation such as a cardiac arrest. Other situations may require us to think carefully and to assimilate new experiences into theoretical knowledge in order to make a decision about the best way forward. Wherever one is working, it is likely to require us to respond in different ways when reasoning through a situation in order to arrive at a relevant decision.

Learning to 'see' mental processes

We have included an Exercise (4.6) that shows a situation from both the perspective of the student nurse and then the mentor, designed to highlight the importance of trying to understand your mentor's mental processes.

Exercise 4.6

The student's experience

At the beginning of your span of duty you enter the bay of patients you are going to be looking after to assess the patient's care needs. Your mentor usually goes to each patient moving from bed one through to bed 6. Today, you are puzzled as, instead of going to the first patient, your mentor goes to a lady who is in bed 4 and asks if she is all right. After a brief conversation with the patient, your mentor finds out that the patient has a terrible migraine that she suffers from periodically (this is unrelated to the reason for her admission). The mentor draws the curtain around the bed, puts a cold compress on the patient's forehead, draws the window blinds, and checks the patient's prescription chart. The mentor then ascertains which medication the patient normally takes for migraine and says she will ask the doctor to prescribe this as soon as possible. She gives the patient the nurse call system and asks the patient to call if she needs anything. The mentor also fetches a vomit bowl for the patient and reassures the patient she will be there if she needs anything.

Think about what the mentor has done.

- List the decisions the mentor has made regarding this patient.
- Which questions would you need to ask the mentor in order to clarify why she has made these decisions?

The mentor's experience

I walked into the bay of patients I was allocated for the day. As usual I scan the patients on entering the bay and noticed the patient in bed 4 didn't look at all well and seemed to be in pain. The other patients looked reasonably comfortable so I decided I needed to find out what was the matter with the lady in bed 4.

As soon as I knew it was a migraine, I closed the curtain and blinds as people are often photosensitive when they have a migraine. I decided to apply a cold compress for comfort and decided to fetch a vomit bowl as migraine can cause nausea and vomiting.

From scanning the prescription chart, there was no medication prescribed for migraine. After finding out what normally works for the patient, I decided to get a prescription from the doctor to try and limit the patient's discomfort.

Pain can often increase if the patient becomes anxious, so I reassured her by giving her the means to call a nurse if she needed one and reassured her that I was on hand should she feel worse or need anything.

This simple scenario helps to highlight the importance of understanding what your mentor is doing. The student is puzzled by the mentor's behaviour in going straight to bed 4. However, the mentor has scanned her patients, picks up cues that all is not well with a specific patient, checks the other patients to make sure her priority is the patient in bed 4, and goes to deal with the patient she feels is her priority at that moment. The mentor has clearly worked through a process that the student cannot see.

The student can learn a lot from the actions that the mentor implements for the patient in bed 4 but, importantly, the student cannot observe the rationales for why the mentor has made a decision to prioritize the lady in bed 4. However, this is an important aspect to learn from the mentor. It is easy to imagine how, in not scanning the patients and picking up on non-verbal cues, the mentor could get sidetracked with the patients in beds 1–3, leaving the patient with the migraine to suffer for a longer period. Should the situation have been more urgent than a migraine, the patient may have suffered other more serious consequences.

This is what is meant by learning to see your mentor's mental processes. It is about asking the right questions. Did you include in your exercise to question the mentor as to why she went to the patient in bed 4 first? Of course it is not always possible or appropriate to question your mentor at the bedside. You need to consider ways in which you maximize your learning and decision making given the very busy environments you find yourself exposed to.

It is quite useful to carry a notebook and jot questions down to ask at a later time, perhaps over a cup of coffee or when you are setting up equipment with your mentor for a specific patient. You may wish to share a reflective account of your experience with your mentor in order to clarify your understanding of why decisions were made. This is quite useful as your perceptions of what has happened may be incorrect due to a lack of knowledge, misinterpretation, or lack of understanding of the bigger picture at the time of the experience. Your mentor is in a prime position to help you learn from these experiences and to clear up any misconceptions that occurred at the time.

Exercise 4.7

You are working with the community nurse who is your mentor. Your mentor says she has a full list and a meeting to attend at 2 p.m. She says she needs to work quickly today. One of the patients you have to visit is an elderly gentleman who has had a stroke, suffers from depression and a loss of appetite. His stroke has left him quite dependent, with an unsteady gait and generalized weakness. You are visiting today to give him his injection of vitamin B12 as he also has pernicious anaemia.

This gentleman lives with his daughter who has given up work to look after him. The daughter seems very quiet and withdrawn, which is not usual for her.

After giving him his injection, your mentor goes to say goodbye to the daughter. The daughter offers you both a cup of tea, which the mentor accepts. Your mentor sits down to have a drink and a chat to the daughter.

Think about why your mentor decides to spend time on this visit when she has said she is really busy.

 What might the consequences be if she does not take the time to do this?

 What might the consequences be of taking this chunk of time out of her day?

 Is the decision to have a cup of tea and a chat the one that you would have made?

Learning to develop reasoning skills and make decisions

We have already identified in Chapter 2 that experience does not equal learning. It is so important to think about the experiences that you have, talk to other members of the team, search the literature to enhance your knowledge about the experiences you have, and reflect on these to identify your future learning needs. As you progress in terms of nursing experience, and begin to manage nursing care, it is useful to identify the reasons that led you to make particular decisions. Verbalizing/documenting your reasoning and discussing these with your mentor help you and your mentor to identify aspects that you need to work on. It may highlight:

- gaps/errors in your reasoning/knowledge
- deficits with regard to your repertoire of skills
- how you have developed in terms of your nursing competence
- reassurance in your developing confidence
- aspects of nursing you need to work at within your placement.

Exercise 4.8

Reflect on a decision you have made during a span of duty. From your reflection, identify your development needs and discuss these with your mentor.

Note: You may wish to use this exercise as a piece of your portfolio evidence.

Remember, experience does not equal learning. Likewise learning does not equal personal development. It is only when you apply your learning to a specific context of your experience that your clinical reasoning and decision making can develop. Other important aspects of your development are your reflective learning and the feedback that you receive from your mentor.

Exercise 4.9

You are involved in caring for a patient, and, while undertaking a review of their health needs, you discover that their blood pressure is very low, and they often feel faint when standing up or getting out of bed in the morning. They are on a variety of medicines for their health problems.

Think about how you would proceed in this situation:

 How would you decide this patient's blood pressure was abnormally low?

 What sort of information would you need to gather?

Which sources of information might you consult?

 With whom might you discuss this patient's problems?

 What decision might be appropriate in this situation?

Reasoning

Reasoning is about asking questions of yourself, seeking out information, deciding on the options available to you, and deciding on the best option utilizing the information available to you. You should then seek out your mentor to present the information and to describe how and why you have reached the decision that you feel is most appropriate. In doing this, you will not only ensure your course of action is an appropriate one in the given situation but this will also allow your mentor to give feedback to you. It also allows your mentor to evaluate your learning, identify at which stage of the decision-making framework you are at, and to give constructive feedback to you if there are pertinent aspects that you have not considered that may alter the options available and hence the decision that you make.

For example, if you go straight to your mentor and say 'I think this patient's blood pressure is low', this will alert the mentor to a potential problem that they can then investigate and this may be appropriate as a very junior student. However, by thinking through what you know of the patient, comparing previous readings with the current one, considering what might have affected their blood pressure, reviewing the medications they are on, reviewing the health problems that they have, and considering possible actions, this demonstrates your previous learning to your mentor and how you are applying your knowledge and experience to new situations. In other words, you are demonstrating reasoning skills and your decision making ability.

Using portfolio evidence to support your practice achievement

In writing down your decisions made from examples such as in Exercise 4.9, you can 'capture' your learning in a written record to provide evidence for your portfolio. This can help the development of your increasing competence in relation to decision-making. In keeping portfolio evidence to demonstrate your decision making ability, it is also useful to read these from time to time to make sure you are continuing to develop. It is also reassuring to be able to review your developing ability, and to identify further developmental needs from your portfolio evidence. Written evidence also assists your mentor in making a judgement about your proficiency as a developing student, and reminds them of your experiences and how you have learned from them.

Mentor feedback – using feedback to enhance your reasoning and decision making skills

A key role of the mentor is to provide both formative and summative feedback to you as a student.

Formative feedback may take the form of:

- some comments on your performance and the decisions you have made while you are working alongside the mentor delivering care
- the fact that your mentor gives you more, or less, responsibility for patient care
- verbal feedback/discussion about how to approach situations differently in the future
- verbal pointers towards further information sources that will increase your knowledge and, if utilized, will inform your future reasoning and decision making.

Summative feedback occurs during your final progress interview where the mentor will also make a summative assessment of the level of competence you have achieved by the end of the placement; this is required as part of your documented progress interviews on completion of the placement.

Actively seeking feedback from your mentor can enhance your development considerably. It also helps your mentor to focus on what you need from them.

It is always easy to give positive feedback on a student's performance but can be much harder to develop the form that constructive feedback will take when as a student you need to work on the skills that you are developing.

Exercise 4.10

Think about your own experiences where your mentor has given you feedback about your performance. Try to identify at least one example of positive feedback and one experience of constructive feedback (you may wish to refer back to your portfolio to refresh your memory).

- What sort of feedback did you receive?
- How did this make you feel?
- Did the feedback identify how your reasoning and your decision making skills were developing?
- Did your mentor help you to identify an action plan for the future to enhance your skills?
- What sort of input did you have into this process?
- How could you gain more from the feedback that you receive in the future?

Receiving feedback from your mentor should contain an account regarding how far you have progressed during your placement as well as what you can do to develop your skills further during future practice experiences. It can be particularly difficult for both the student and the mentor when the feedback is less positive than was hoped for from previous discussions. This can make the mentor anxious about giving feedback, and the student can feel upset and perhaps angry at the comments that they hear. Alternatively, feedback can be a great motivator to learn. This may be because of very positive comments about your progress that make you want to do even better, or the student can become more motivated to develop their skills as they realize they have not quite made the progress that was anticipated but have an action plan to address the identified issues.

If your mentor did not refer to your clinical reasoning and decision making skills, make a note to address this particular aspect the next time you meet with your mentor. The biggest difference between a health care support worker and a registered nurse is that the nurse needs not only to perform nursing care, he or she needs to interpret information, make sound judgements, and use their reasoning skills to make effective decisions in their professional capacity.

Of course, if the feedback is less positive, this can also demotivate you as a learner. You may think it is pointless continuing on your programme of study. Try to stand back from what has been said. This may take some time to be able to do this. Ask yourself some questions, or discuss what was said with someone whom you can trust (this may be a friend, another colleague, or your personal tutor). Think about:

 What was actually said?

 Is there any basis for the mentor saying this?

 What can you do to improve your performance/deal with the issues?

Taking positive action may not make you feel better about yourself straight away but it will give you a positive focus, and will give you the opportunity to develop your potential.

You need to be an active participant in your learning and take responsibility for this. It will also give you a greater sense of achievement when your mentor can give you positive feedback on your progress and development. It may help to reflect on what competence consists of, that is, knowledge, skills and professional values.

Learning from experience and storytelling

You can learn much from listening to the stories that other nurses and health care professionals tell, as storytelling is a way of teaching and learning that existed even before the development of written language (Yoder-Wise and Kowalski, 2003). Stories are accounts that create memorable pictures in the mind of the listener (Sorrell and Redmond, 2002) and I am sure that we can all recount stories that we heard a long time ago with incredible detail.

The stories that nurses tell can be used to interpret health care, by exploring the lived experience of nurses, their patients and their families (Ahlberg and Gibson, 2003). Stories can also give a tremendous insight into how culture can impact on decision making, and can engender the art of listening in students (Schwarz and Abbott, 2007). Stories also contextualize and humanize knowledge; they deal with the know-how of nursing (Benner, 1984) that is so essential to skilled practice (Bowles, 1995).

Stories can also help to develop critical thinking (Davidhizar and Lonser, 2003) and are an effective way of transmitting knowledge and promoting problem-solving (Schwarz and Abbott, 2007).

What is evident from the relevant literature is that storytelling can be a rich and informative source from which we can learn. However, we have to develop our listening skills and reflect on the stories that we are told in order to gain insight from others' experiences, and thus learn from these stories. Most nurses tell stories about their experiences and so your mentor may be a rich source of information through the stories they tell. Listening to these stories that often detail both successes that individuals have achieved, as well as the mistakes they have made, can be a tremendous learning experience without having to live through the pain and frustration of negative events (Yoder-Wise and Kowalski, 2003).

Exercise 4.11   A story told

When I was a first-year student (I think it was my second placement), I was asked to go and help out on another ward as they were extremely busy. The ward sister asked me to help her with the drug round. As we went round with the medicines, I noticed that lots of patients were dressed in their own clothes and very few had identification bracelets on them.

Sister asked me to take some tablets into Mr Singh in the side room. She informed me that he would need a beaker to drink from as he had had a stroke and his hands were a bit shaky.

I went into the sideroom and asked the gentleman sitting by the bed if he was Mr Singh, to which he said yes. I poured Mr Singh some water into a beaker so he could take his tablets. Mr Singh took the tablets.

When I went back to the ward sister, I suggested Mr Singh's condition must have improved a lot as he didn't seem to need a beaker to drink from.

It was only then that I realized I had given the tablets to Mr Singh's visitor and he had taken them! I nearly left nursing because of this. It was so embarrassing and so stupid.

In reading this story, think about the following questions:

- **(?)** What is your response to the story?
- **(?)** Which mistakes were made?
- **(?)** What can be learned from this story?
- **(?)** How might it influence your practice and the decisions you make in the future?

We can learn not only from our own experiences but can also learn from the stories people tell. This can be a powerful method of learning. In particular, if we can recognize the inappropriate decisions made in particular situations, this is a safe way of learning. Hopefully, it will also help you to prevent disasters in your decision making in similar situations in the future.

Conclusion

The role that your mentor plays in helping you to develop clinical reasoning and decision making is a vital part of your education programme and your development. Take the time to think about how you can get the most out of your mentor in order to maximize your personal development.

References

Ahlberg, K. and Gibson, F. (2003) 'What is the story telling us'?: using patient experiences to improve practice, *European Journal of Oncology Nursing*, 7(3): 149–50.

Benner, P. (1984) *From Novice to Expert: Power and Excellence in Clinical Nursing*. Menlo Park, CA: Jossey-Bass.

Bowles, N. (1995) Storytelling: a search for meaning within nursing practice, *Nurse Education Today*, 15: 365–9.

Clarke, C. L., Gibb, C. E. and Ramprogus, B. (2003) Clinical learning environments: an evaluation of an innovative role to support preregistration nursing placements, *Learning in Health and Social Care*, 2(2): 105–15.

Davidhizar, R. and Lonser, G. (2003) Storytelling as a teaching technique, *Nurse Educator* 28(5): 217–21.

Davies, C., Welham, V., Glover, A., Jones, L. and Murphy, F. (1999) Teaching in practice, *Nursing Standard*, 13(35): 33–8.

Driscoll, J. (1994) Reflective practice for practise – a framework of structured reflection for clinical areas, *Senior Nurse*, 14(1): 47–50.

Honey, P. and Mumford, A. (1992) *The Manual of Learning Styles*. Maidenhead: Peter Honey Publications.

Neary, M. (1997) Defining the role of assessors, mentors and supervisors: part 1, *Nursing Standard*, 11(42): 34–9.

Nursing and Midwifery Council (NMC) (2008) *Standards to Support Learning and Assessment in Practice*. London: NMC.

Philips, R. M., Davies, W.B. and Neary, M. (1996) The practitioner teacher: a study of the introduction of mentors in the pre-registration nurse education programme in Wales: part 2, *Journal of Advanced Nursing*, 23: 1080–8.

Schwarz, M. and Abbott, A. (2007) Storytelling: a clinical application for undergraduate nursing students, *Nurse Education in Practice*, 7: 181–6.

Sharples, K. (2009) *Learning to Learn in Nursing Practice*, 1st edn. Exeter: Learning Matters Ltd.

Sorrell, J. and Redmond, G. (2002) *Community-based Nursing Practice: Learning Through Students' Stories*. Philadelphia, PA: FA Davis.

Spouse, J. (1996) The effective mentor: a model for student centred learning in clinical practice, *Nursing Times Research*, 1: 120–33.

Spouse, J. (2001) Bridging theory and practice in the supervisory relationship: a sociocultural perspective, *Journal of Advanced Nursing*, 33(4): 512–22.

Yoder-Wise, P. and Kowalski, K. (2003) The power of storytelling, *Nursing Outlook*, 51: 37–42.

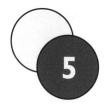

5 Making decisions as part of a team

- **Introduction**
- **What is a team?**
- **Being part of a nursing team**
- **Communication in teams**
- **Being part of a multiprofessional team**
- **What makes an effective team?**
- **Decision making in the multiprofessional team**
- **Conclusion**
- **References**

Introduction

Within nursing you not only learn from your mentor but also from being part of a team, often a multiprofessional team. As such it is important to build relationships with the whole team and learn to work as an effective member of the team. In this chapter we explore what makes an effective team, how we learn to be part of a team, learn from the team, and how working effectively as a team member can aid your clinical reasoning and decision making.

There are difficulties in defining what a team is. In relation to health care, we talk about nursing teams, midwifery teams, as well as the multiprofessional team. For the purpose of this chapter, we focus first on the nursing team followed by exploring the multiprofessional team, and how the team can aid us in developing our decision-making processes. We have already discussed in Chapter 2 how reflection can help us to learn from our experience, from Chapter 3 about portfolio work and how this can help you to learn from experience; this can be further developed within this chapter. Learning from the experience of teamwork is useful in developing your knowledge, accessing other health care profession's skills and expertise, and contributing specific nursing/midwifery expertise in helping others to learn from effective teamwork experiences.

What is a team?

A team is not just a group of people who happen to work in the same field or vicinity; that is, within the health care system. A team is more than just a group. Clark (2008) identifies some key elements of teamwork:

- interdependence
- common goals/tasks
- commitment to each other
- personal growth
- synergy
- co-operation
- shared management functions.

A key element here is synergy. This means that any individual can be effective in what they specifically do for an individual. However, with regard to a group of professionals fulfilling their individual roles, when they work as a team they can produce a degree of effectiveness for an individual patient/client group that adds up to more than the numbers of individual tasks that are involved. In short, they provide holistic, person-centred care that is seamless and which results in enhanced quality of care, catering for the total needs of a patient/client group.

Mohrman et al. (1995) define a team as 'a group of individuals who work together to produce products or deliver services for which they are mutually accountable'. There is substantial evidence that teamwork can lead to increased effectiveness in terms of both the quality and quantity of services delivered (Guzzo and Shea, 1992; Weldon and Weingart, 1993).

There is no consensus on the number of individuals who are necessary to make up a team and it is also difficult to define a team as there appears to be no specific recipe as to what makes a team. It is more about the processes within a team that make it successful or not. However, a team needs to be small enough to enable it to function in the way Clark (2008) describes, but large enough to fulfil their roles in terms of increased effectiveness for patients/clients.

In terms of a group, you might belong to a group of people undertaking an aerobics class and, while you have a shared goal, that is, keeping fit, you do not need to work together in order to do this. How fit you become will be a measure of the individual effort you put into the exercises, and the outcome is not dependent on others working with you. However, if you belong to a football or netball team, there is a shared goal but, in addition, the success of your team will depend on how all players work together, and trust and respect for the individual roles that members play are often vital in terms of predicting success or not. There is also evidence in health care that effective teamwork contributes to increased efficiency, access to services and quality of patient care (West, 1999), with Borrill et al. (2000) describing how teamwork among health professionals increases both job satisfaction and the mental health of team members.

Hence, it can be seen how important effective teamwork is for all team members as well as the individuals the team is providing care for. When you start to learn about nursing, a key element is to learn how to function as part of the nursing/midwifery team as well as how be effective as part of the broader multiprofessional health care team.

Exercise 5.1

Think of the groups and teams you are part of in a personal and professional capacity. Make a list of these.

Can you identify from thinking about how those groups and teams function what the differences are between a group and a team?

Groups	Teams

Being part of a nursing team

Exercise 5.2

(?) What is your role within the nursing team?

(?) What can you contribute?

(?) What can you learn from the team?

What is your role in the nursing team?	What can you contribute to the team?	What can you learn from the team?

The role of a student in learning to be a nurse or midwife must be to first acquire some specialist knowledge, relevant professional skills, and the professional approach and attitudes necessary to be able to function effectively as a nurse/midwife. Initially, as a student your role is to actively seek out opportunities to learn about your intended profession, thus demonstrating commitment to your profession. As you progress throughout your course, you begin to make more active contributions within the team to patient care delivery, to share your experience and knowledge with others and ultimately to contribute to decision making within the team. As a team member, you need to get to know the philosophy of the team you are working with in order to understand what the team's goals and aspirations are. You may do this through attending team meetings and reading the placement's philosophy of care as well as through talking to team members. You also need to demonstrate that the team can trust you to be conscientious in what they ask you to do, and to seek help when unsure.

What you can learn from the team can be limitless but may include:

- specialist knowledge and skills
- different approaches to teamwork
- roles of team members
- what makes a good/not so good team
- how you might develop your teamwork skills
- what sort of leader you might like to be
- how to develop a team.

Exercise 5.3

Your mentor asks you to stay with a post-operative patient, Mrs Brown, whose condition is unstable at the moment. She asks you to monitor this patient closely and record half-hourly observations of pulse, temperature, respirations and blood pressure and to alert her if the patient's observations alter (she gives you parameters to work within). While you are with the patient, another staff nurse asks you to come immediately and help her to wash a patient. You try to tell her that your mentor has asked you to stay with this patient but she tells you not to argue, she was not aware of this, and to come with her.

Later, your mentor is quite cross with you as the half-hourly observations haven't been done on Mrs Brown.

What are your thoughts about how the team has functioned in this situation?

You may have included some of the following points:

- good communication from your mentor
- poor communication skills demonstrated by the second staff nurse
- poor communication between team members about both the patient and the role assigned to you
- this team appears to have a hierarchical structure
- reduced efficiency and safety in terms of patient care
- the importance of being listened to as a student
- the importance of assertiveness when working within a team.

Communication in teams

Effective communication is the essence of a good team and this scenario demonstrates how poor communication can result in patients being put at risk. All team members need to be listened to and respected. It can be particularly difficult as a student to be assertive. However, you do need to learn to be assertive in situations such as these in order to protect the patient from harm. Two decisions were made by the student in this example. The first decision was not to pursue communicating why he or she needed to remain with Mrs Brown. The student's second decision was to decide to go with the staff nurse to wash another patient. Both decisions made could have had a detrimental effect on the patient who required half-hourly monitoring.

Being part of a multiprofessional team

Your role within the multiprofessional team is similar to that of the nursing team but involves learning about other health care disciplines, the roles they play within the team and how these roles interact and complement the care a person receives in order for the patient/client to receive efficient and effective health care.

Exercise 5.4

List the members who make up the multiprofessional team.

You might have included the following:

- nurses/midwives
- medical staff

- physiotherapists
- occupational therapists
- housekeeping staff
- domestic assistants
- health care support workers
- social workers
- chaplaincy staff
- receptionist/administrative staff
- managers.

It is important to learn about and recognize the contributions that everyone within the team makes as effective working of all members contributes to the overall experience and outcome for the patient. Learning about everyone's roles will aid your clinical reasoning and decision making as you become knowledgeable about the resources available within the team and the limits you have to work within.

The importance of multiprofessional, interprofessional and interagency working has been highlighted in health and social care policy (DoH, 1996, 1997, 2000) with an emphasis on teamwork as a means of ensuring the most effective and efficient provision of health and social care (Cook et al., 2001). Communication is the key to effective decision making within the mutiprofessional team. However, there can be some potential disadvantages when making decisions about patient/client care.

Exercise 5.5

What do you think the potential disadvantages are of working in a multi-professional team?

Potential disadvantages may include:

- personality clashes
- professional clashes
- hierarchical role structures in a team
- a dilution of individual professional responsibility for patients/clients.

Source: Robinson and Wiles (1994).

Exercise 5.6

What can hinder your contribution to:

- the nursing team?
- the multiprofessional team?

Use the table to complete the exercise.

Nursing team	Multiprofessional team

Your answers to this activity may have been similar for both types of team. When working in a team the student may feel their contribution is hindered by some of the following points:

- lack of confidence
- lack of professional knowledge and expertise
- not knowing the patients well enough
- not feeling valued as a student
- hierarchical structures within the team
- poor communication within the team
- previous negative experiences of working in a team
- not understanding the roles of team members.

What makes an effective team?

Effective communication is the fundamental key in relation to any kind of team. In order to attain this all team members must feel valued for their contribution and respected within the team. Where there is a hierarchical structure, this will affect the confidence of team members to contribute, discuss and challenge assumptions made. Individuals who feel valued and respected will be able to develop their knowledge of each team member's role as they will feel able to ask questions without feeling inadequate.

Developing knowledge

Developing an in-depth knowledge of the patients you are working with will enable you to increase your contribution to team decisions. Without an in-depth knowledge, your ability to contribute to decisions made will be less effective and may be contrary to the best interests of the patient and their significant others. Developing your nursing knowledge and expertise will also aid your contribution to the team, particularly if it is based on sound theoretical knowledge and experience.

Reflecting on experiences

As a student you need to learn as much as you can from the experiences you are exposed to. Reflecting on your experiences and developing action plans (as discussed in Chapter 2) will help you to develop a significant body of knowledge and experience that will enhance your contribution to team processes. Reflection on poor experiences in teams and planning your future actions will also help you to develop confidence to contribute to the team. The important aspect is to learn from both positive and less positive experiences and to develop an action plan that will help you to increase your confidence in the future.

Consider the following activity (Exercise 5.7).

Exercise 5.7

An elderly lady is admitted to a medical ward. She is extremely breathless, has a chesty cough, a high temperature and is thought to be suffering from pneumonia. She normally has limited mobility and is only able to walk a few steps using a walking frame. Currently, she is confined to bed as she feels too weak to get out of bed. She has also suffered with urinary incontinence for the last few months and as a result has been reluctant to drink much.

Which health care professionals might be involved in this lady's care?

You may have considered the following:

- nurses
- doctors
- physiotherapist
- support staff
- administrative staff
- domestic staff.

Who makes which decisions in the team?

The sort of care and decisions that may be involved in this lady's care may be:

Nurse

- vital signs observations will be made and a decision made as to how frequent they need to be depending on the findings
- a nursing assessment will be undertaken to identify nursing needs that will need to be addressed
- appropriate positioning for a breathless patient
- pressure risk assessment due to mobility problem and appropriate aids utilized
- provision of a sputum pot for a specimen
- moving and handling assessment with referral to the physiotherapist
- urinalysis and continence assessment, with appropriate actions implemented
- commence a fluid intake and output chart
- decision on the level of support required for hygiene needs
- monitoring of bowel function due to limited mobility and possible reduced fluid intake
- nutritional monitoring due to breathlessness
- administer prescribed medicines.

Doctor

- examination of the patient and a medical history to identify the potential/most likely diagnosis
- request sputum specimen
- request a chest X-ray
- prescribe antibiotics.

Physiotherapist

- in-depth mobility assessment
- advice to nursing staff
- decision on the most appropriate mobility aid.

Support staff

- Support staff will often be the individual who delivers a lot of the essential care such as hygiene, feeding, toileting, giving fluids, taking observations, and so on. They make decisions about what they will feed back to you in terms of how the patient is coping with these activities.

Administrative staff

- ensures patient information is inputted into the organization administrative processes

- organizes requests for investigations and transport of specimens to the laboratories
- orders transport
- ensures the smooth running of the placement by answering telephones, taking messages and requests from staff.

Domestic staff

- often responsible for delivering food and fluids to the patient and removing trays and water jugs
- feed back to nursing staff about how much the patient is eating and drinking
- clean beds and patient areas to reduce the incidence of hospital acquired infection.

Exercise 5.8

How does each health care professional's role complement other's roles within the team?

Each member of the different professions has a specific role to play in ensuring this patient has the best opportunity of getting well and preventing further problems occurring. The nurses' role is to help this person fulfil their daily living activities and to prevent further problems such as dehydration. The doctor's role is to diagnose and treat specific problems. The physiotherapist assesses mobility and needs to work closely with the nursing staff to ensure moving and handling decisions are continued. The support staff deliver most of the daily care with domestic staff ensuring food and fluids are distributed to the patient. The administrative staff ensures the patient's investigations are undertaken promptly by ensuring request forms are dealt with appropriately.

Exercise 5.9

Using an example from your current experience or from your portfolio work through a similar activity that is relevant to your own branch of nursing or midwifery.

Exercise 5.10

What might potentially happen if team members did not work together?

You may have considered that at the very least the patient's treatment and/or discharge might be delayed. However, there could be more serious problems. For example, if the nurse made a decision not to give the patient their medicines because the patient said they did not want them and the nurse chose to respect that decision without following it up to find out why or reporting it. You need to note from this example that even making no decision is a decision that can have consequences for the patient and the nurse.

Decision making in the multiprofessional team

Using your branch experience to inform decision making, consider the relevant scenario from the following examples in Example 5.11. Using these examples you can practise highlighting the range of decisions you may be required to make within specific branches of nursing. It will be useful before you start this exercise to refer back to the decision making framework introduced in Chapter 1 to identify the stage you are at and what is expected of you in terms of decision making. We will recap it here.

1st stage of decision making

You gain experience, gather information, reflect on what you know or might need to know, and discuss with your mentor what might be needed in a given situation to begin to increase your repertoire of knowledge and decision making. At this stage your mentor is your key reference point before taking action.

2nd stage of decision making

At this stage you have gained some experience and should have learned a lot from the mentors you have worked with. You should be able to apply past experience and theoretical knowledge to new experiences to be able to discuss with your mentor the decisions that might be appropriate in a given situation. Your mentor will act as a guide to the most appropriate decisions, but you will be starting to demonstrate that you can utilize your own initiative within situations that are similar to those you have encountered before.

3rd stage of decision making

Within the 3rd stage, you should now have a wealth of experience from a variety of placements. In addition, you should be fairly knowledgeable about local policies and procedures, as well as having built up considerable knowledge regarding best available evidence, and how it can be applied to your own branch of nursing and midwifery. Your mentor will still be your point of reference but, at this stage, you should be making decisions fairly independently, only needing to verify that your mentor agrees that your decision is appropriate within the given situation.

Exercise 5.11

Read through the scenarios below and select one to work on that relates to your experience.

Using your chosen scenario:

- Apply the 'add on framework' of decision making, appropriate to the relevant point of your course, consider the nursing decisions you will make in the situation.
- Consider the other members of the multiprofessional team you might decide the patient needs referral to, giving an explanation for why the referral is relevant, that is, you need to justify the decision/s that you make.
- You may wish to discuss your decisions with your peers, your personal tutor, or your mentor to access others' experience and views on the decisions made.

Adult branch

John, aged 72, has been referred to the district nursing team. He has had repeated chest infections and is breathless most of the time. He has been a smoker for over 50 years and has previously been diagnosed with chronic obstructive pulmonary disease (COPD). John lives by himself and has been quite 'down' for a long time. He is finding it increasingly difficult to manage at home and the GP is concerned about how he is coping.

When you meet John, he seems very withdrawn, he is rather emaciated, and there is a lack of eye contact. He is very breathless and is coughing a lot. While he sounds very chesty, he is not able to cough any sputum up. There is a rather full ashtray beside him.

Learning disabilities

Jack, aged 20, who has mild learning disabilities, has been referred to your day care facility to help him with daily life care skills. Ros, his key community worker, has requested this referral particularly as he appears to be contracting repeated attacks of diarrhoea that she believes to be as a result of not washing his hands properly.

When Jack arrives at your unit, he seems withdrawn and is quite unkempt. His mother has accompanied him. Jack's mother also says she is extremely worried about him and is really fed up that he won't respond to or act on her advice.

Mental health

Maria, aged 26, has been referred to your mental health inpatient facility because of a recent self-harming episode (she took an overdose of tablets). She has herself agreed to be admitted and has come to your unit accompanied by her husband, Dave.

Letter of referral

Thank you for agreeing to admit this lady who has recently been in our care for treatment of a paracetamol overdose. This was dealt with successfully and, from a physical point of view, she has no further problems. We do know from her brief stay in our department that she has recently had some personal problems which may have led to this episode. Neither Maria nor her husband were willing to discuss these with us at that stage.

Child branch

Lisa, a 4-year-old, has been admitted to your unit. She is accompanied by her mother who is extremely anxious. Lisa is crying and irritable, and now has a temperature of 38.5. Lisa's mother is also anxious as she has two other children who will be returning from school later this afternoon and she has no one to meet the children at school.

Letter from GP about Lisa

Thank you for admitting this 4-year-old child whom I saw today in my surgery. She has a history of fever (38°C) for 24 hours and her mother thinks she may have had a febrile convulsion earlier today but cannot confirm this. I suspect that she may have a viral illness as, according to her mother, some other children at her nursery have had something similar. I am asking for her to be admitted to monitor the situation.

Midwifery

Lisa is 6 months pregnant and is a single mother. She attends your antenatal clinic and is very distressed. Her blood pressure is elevated and her ankles are quite swollen. While talking to her she discloses that she has found out her boyfriend is seeing someone else and he has left their rented flat. She has no contact with her family and they live quite far away. She is really worried about what will happen to her and where she is going to live as she can't afford the rent on her flat.

Lisa is adamant that she doesn't want to contact her family as she is sure they wouldn't want anything to do with her. She says she has a terrible headache and really doesn't want to go through with this pregnancy now.

Conclusion

From working through this chapter, you should be aware of how teamwork is an essential component of health care work. If we are to deliver effective care for our patients/service users, we need to ensure that we develop good communication systems, be aware of each other's primary roles, work collaboratively in order to support each other, and be aware of the potential effect that the decisions we make have on others within the team, as well as on the patient/client.

As a health professional, you need to utilize resources to maximum effect and enlist the assistance of the most appropriate health care professionals. In addition, through being aware of the importance of the roles that team members fulfil, you will recognize other people's value within health care delivery, and should develop respect for the expertise of others that contributes to successful care delivery. Inattention to the roles team members fulfil, and a lack of awareness of the contribution that others make, will result in potential care deficits that can affect the quality of care delivered and the success of the outcome for an individual.

References

Borrill, C., West, M., Shapiro, D. and Rees, A. (2000) Teamworking and effectiveness in healthcare, *British Journal of Healthcare Management*, 6(8): 364–71.

Clark, D. (2008) Cited in B. Goodman and R. Clemow (2008) *Nursing and Working with Other People*, Chapter 6, p. 140. Exeter: Learning Matters Ltd.

Cook, G., Gerrish, K. and Clarke, C. (2001) Decision making in teams: issues arising from two evaluations, *Journal of Interprofessional Care*, 2(2): 141–51.

Department of Health (DoH) (1996) *Primary Care: Delivering the Future*. London: Her Majesty's Stationery Office (HMSO).

Department of Health (DoH) (1997) *Developing Partnerships in Mental Health*. Wetherby: Her Majesty's Stationery Office (HMSO).

Department of Health (DoH) (2000) *The NHS Plan: A Plan for Investment, A Plan for Reform*. London: Her Majesty's Stationery Office (HMSO).

Guzzo, R.A. and Shea, G.P. (1992) Cited in C. Borrill, M. West, D. Shapiro and A. Reese (2000) Teamworking and effectiveness in healthcare, *British Journal of Healthcare Management*, 6(8): 364–71.

Mohrma, S.A., Cohen, S.G. and Mohrman, A.M. Jr (1995) *Designing Team Based Organisations*. San Francisco, CA: Jossey-Bass.

Robinson, J. and Wiles R. (1994) *Teamwork in Primary Health Care: Do Patients Benefit?* Southampton: Institution for Health Policy Studies.

Weldon, E. and Weingart, L.R. (1993) Group goals and group performance, *British Journal of Social Psychology*, 32: 307–34.

West, M. (1999) Communication and teamworking in healthcare, *Nursing Times Research*, 4(1): 8–17.

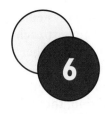

6 Ethical and legal issues in decision making

- **Introduction**
- **Beginning to manage a patient's care**
- **Targets for care**
- **Legal and ethical issues**
- **Ethical decision making**
- **Moral and ethical dilemmas**
- **Prioritizing care**
- **Ethical decisions within the team**
- **Legal issues in nursing**
- **Consent to treatment and care**
- **Being reasonably informed**
- **Consent**
- **Duty of care**
- **Documentation**
- **Handing information over to other staff**
- **Conclusion**
- **References**

Introduction

Chapter 5 guided you through functioning as a team member and you will no doubt already have begun to be involved in decision making in consultation with other members of the health care team (both nursing and multiprofessional). The purpose of this chapter is to take you forward a stage where you will begin to make decisions about managing patients, considering some of the ethical and legal issues involved in so doing.

Beginning to manage a patient's care

Beginning to manage patient care means that your clinical practice will be assessed on Bondy Level 3. At this level of practice, you will be in the second year of your pre-registration course. What do you believe to be the differences in practice between a first and second-year student?

Stage 1

At Stage 1 of the 'add on framework' you are learning a repertoire of nursing skills under direct supervision, and are starting to reflect on your practice. In addition, while learning how to undertake specific skills for patients, you should be starting to read the relevant policies and procedure that will guide your practice, you will be learning from your mentor about the decisions that are made in a particular situation, and beginning to increase your knowledge of nursing by reading about different topics.

Stage 2

At Stage 2 of the 'add on framework', you will have acquired essential nursing skills and be able to practise them safely. You will also start to be able to apply specific guidelines in the policies and procedures that you can adapt according to the situation that you are in. At this stage you should also be able to articulate the rationales for why you have suggested a particular course of action from your increasing knowledge of nursing. In addition, as you start to manage patient care, you will be exposed to dilemmas that nurses face every day.

You will find it useful to reflect on the transition from Stage 1 to Stage 2 in the 'add on framework' for inclusion as a portfolio entry.

In considering nursing, Vestal (2008) has described the work of nursing as: 'a complex web of people, processes and technology' (p. 8) and requires the nurse to 'constantly respond to arising issues' (p. 8).

It can be deduced from the above quote that managing the work of nursing is hugely different from managing an industrial process. There has been a temptation in recent years to try and apply industrial management systems to the work of nursing. Management techniques (of which industry has a long history) have not always been evident in nursing. However, properly applied and adapted for nursing, these can result in better patient care and effective and efficient use of scarce resources.

Targets for care

The introduction of targets for care is but one example of the application of management systems into health care. The introduction of a four-hour target for emergency department (ED) waiting times for treatment means that patients are seen and dealt with in the ED very quickly.

However, meeting these four-hour targets means that a person either needs to be discharged from ED within a four-hour period, or a bed for in-patient treatment must be found. Finding a bed to treat a person as an in-patient can then impact on nurses in other areas who may have to discharge other patients from their wards, or move their patients to another area so they can accommodate the needs of the patient from ED.

This can pose particular ethical dilemmas for a nurse especially if the only patient who can move to another area is elderly and confused. Moving areas could confuse and disorientate this patient further, thus causing potential harm to an individual. However, not accepting a patient from ED could impact on other individuals in the ED that are still waiting to be treated as there is not the space to do so until a patient is transferred out of the department. This leads to an ethical dilemma, and difficult decisions have to be made sometimes. Frameworks that can be applied to such dilemmas in order to assist your decision making in a case such as this will be discussed shortly.

Legal and ethical issues

You will probably have noticed that as you progress from a first- to a second-year student that you begin to draw more on previous experiences when making your care decisions. You will also begin to discuss more with your peers and supervisors aspects of decision making (see the 'add on framework' – 2nd Stage). These strategies will certainly come to the fore when you begin to consider ethical and legal aspects of decision making. There are now numerous texts in the fields of ethics and legal aspects of nursing care and it is not the remit of this text to replicate a large amount of this material. However, the Nursing and Midwifery Council (NMC) in *The Code: Standards of Conduct, Performance and Ethics for Nurses and Midwives* (2008) do set out very clearly what is expected of qualified nurses and midwives in the way of ethics and legal issues. A later publication from the NMC (2009), *Guidance for the Care of Older People*, expands on *The Code* and offers good advice on how to make ethical decisions. As a student nurse, you must adopt these standards in preparation for qualification.

Ethical decision making

When considering ethical decision making *per se*, Tschudin (2003: 107) makes the point that: 'ethics is not something intellectual and complicated; it is something everyday and practice' and that: 'In most decision making situations it is necessary to consider how problems arise, what they are and what can be done about them' (p. 108).

In considering how legal and ethical issues affect decision making, the nurse has to consider how to act in the patient's best interests. The NMC (2008) make this very clear in *The Code* and state that 'You must respect and support people's rights to accept or decline treatment and care' and 'You must uphold people's rights to be fully involved in decisions about their care.'

However, this can be problematic in everyday practice as there are often situations where it can be difficult to know whether we are truly acting in the patient's best interests. Fullbrook (2007) has previously highlighted the difficulty of knowing what is best for a patient. There can be conflicting beliefs and attitudes between the nurse and the patient. People have different views and ideas of the world. Your values may not be the same as a patient/client or their significant others. Many factors influence an individual's beliefs and attitudes such as cultural background, religion and past experience. Other elements may also influence ethical decisions. These may be:

- patient's relatives/family
- other professions
- organizational policies and resources
- occasionally legal rulings.

Moral and ethical dilemmas

The word 'moral' refers to what a person believes is right (Griffith and Tengnah, 2008) and moral dilemmas occur when there are choices to be made regarding two unsatisfactory alternatives. In addition, in ambiguous situations, it can also be difficult to predict the consequences of your actions (Llewellyn and Hayes, 2008), particularly if you are working with limited information about the whole picture. However, there is guidance available to you when considering ethical dilemmas.

There are five ethical principles to guide us in decision making where moral dilemmas occur; these principles are the value of:

- life
- goodness and rightness
- justice and fairness
- truth-telling and honesty
- individual freedom.

Source: Thiroux and Krasemann (2007).

For the nurse, value of life is about enhancing health and well-being. Goodness and rightness relate to doing good and what is right. Justice and fairness are about equality and, in terms of nursing, treating all patients equally and protecting them from incompetent practice. Truth-telling and honesty relate to being transparent and treating a patient with respect in terms of giving them adequate information. Individual freedom relates to an individual having a choice and being able to make their own choice.

With regard to being faced with two equally unsatisfactory alternatives in situations, frameworks can be applied that can assist in decision making. They will not solve the dilemma for you but do offer some guiding principles that you can utilize to reach your decision. These are:

- respect for autonomy (the rights of the individual)
- non-maleficence (the obligation not to harm others)
- beneficence (the need to promote the well-being of others)
- justice (the obligation to treat others fairly).

Source: Beauchamp and Childress (1989).

Consider a mother who is a smoker who has a child with severe asthma. If the mother continues to smoke in front of her child, she is harming the child who becomes a passive smoker. If the child has asthma, inhaling cigarette smoke will cause further asthma symptoms, and may precipitate a life-threatening situation. You may feel the choice is very simple here in terms of talking to the mother about the dangers of smoking and how to stop smoking. However, the mother says she cannot give up smoking as she becomes extremely irritable when she tries and has hit the child when she has tried to stop smoking previously. In addition, she says smoking helps her cope with her situation, and gives her something for herself when her partner is abusive towards her.

In terms of autonomy, both the mother and child have rights. However, you also should not harm others and it may be detrimental to the mother if you try to insist on her giving up smoking and may cause other harm to the child if she is beaten by the mother. However, the child's well-being is harmed by the passive smoking but the mother's well-being may also be harmed as this is her coping mechanism with her situation. In order to try and be fair to both parties, what could you advise?

You might be able to reach a satisfactory outcome here if you can persuade the mother to smoke only outdoors, away from the child. This allows the mother autonomy and may protect her well-being at this point in time, while protecting the child from harm due to passive smoking.

Think about what ethical principles and the framework you can use to assist your decision making in completing Exercise 6.1. How would you decide what may be in the patient's best interests in the following situations:

Exercise 6.1

Ann is a 16-year-old who has given birth in hospital. The baby was unplanned and the father has not been involved with Ann since. She has been well supported by her immediate family. Both the midwives and the family are very keen for her to breastfeed the baby because there are health benefits for the baby, but Ann is adamant that she is not going to do this since it will tie her down, ruin her social life with her friends and badly affect her body image. You are undertaking an experience on a postnatal ward and Ann seems to have 'latched on' to you as a friend. She confesses that she feels distressed because 'everyone is against her' because she will not breastfeed.

- What are the options for acting in Ann's and the baby's best interests here?
- What are the ethical issues surrounding this scenario?

Often, when resources are restricted and in some cases overtly rationed, it is the case that ethical conflicts arise. Issues constantly arise in areas such as in-vitro fertilization

(IVF) and drug treatments for certain types of cancer. You may wish to consider an example of one of these decisions and reflect on 'both sides of the argument' for a portfolio entry.

Prioritizing care

In managing a person's care, you may be faced with ethical and moral dilemmas in terms of how to prioritize care for that person. For example, a porter might be waiting to take a patient to a specific department for an investigation and needs to hurry as he has other patients that are urgent that he needs to collect. However, your patient is in pain and movement is painful for this person. Your patient has been waiting some time to have this investigation done. You call the investigation unit and they say if this is not undertaken now, the patient may not have this investigation for several days. What might you do in this situation?

This is a difficult dilemma. You want to do no further harm to this person but realize that further harm may occur in the longer term if the investigation is not undertaken now as it may delay vital treatment for this person. You might wish to explain the situation to the patient who, if they are able, can be in a position to make the decision. It would also be useful here to consult your mentor who will be able to advise what might be a way forward in terms of solving this dilemma. There are often no easy answers to situations like this.

Exercise 6.2

Imagine the situation where you have just commenced a shift on your hospital ward. There are six ladies in the bay; it is the first time you have met these patients and all but one of them are very happy and engage with you immediately. They are glad to see you as they are ready for their wash as they have had breakfast. There is, however, one patient in the far corner who is sitting on the side of her bed with her back to both yourself and the other patients. She appears to be very withdrawn and non-communicative.

Which patient would you decide to go to first in this bay of patients?

If you decide to go to the withdrawn patient first, it is likely that you are going to have to spend quite a large proportion of your time at a point where there are likely to be many pressures to 'get tasks done' for the other patients. However, what is the right decision ethically and morally and, importantly, what will demonstrate caring? Do you decide to organize and settle the other ladies with their washes first, deciding that you will talk to the withdrawn lady much later when everything has been completed for the others? Do you decide to quickly go round the other patients first and then to the apparently withdrawn patient? Do you go straight to this withdrawn lady to find out what the issues are? This sort of situation frequently poses a dilemma for the nurse.

It can often be easiest to sort out the needs of those patients who are able to articulate their needs easily. You may also feel the other staff might think you are avoiding work by taking time to talk to your withdrawn patient. However, is it right to respond to the more forthright patients when it appears there is an issue that may be more important that is concerning the quiet, withdrawn patient?

There are no easy answers in this case but, as a nurse, you need to be aware of why you go to some patients first and need to make sure it is not because you are avoiding what might turn out to be a difficult situation with the withdrawn patient.

The best option may be to ask for some help, stating you need to spend some time with the withdrawn patient and so would appreciate someone giving you some support with the other patients.

Exercise 6.3

Now take the situation where you are working on a busy ward that is short-staffed. What do you decide to do in the following situation where events are occurring simultaneously?

- An elderly patient is wandering around the ward and trying to get outside.
- A female patient is confined to bed and has been incontinent of urine.
- A patient needs to be prepared for a cardiac catheterization – she is first on the list.

What do you do for the best here? Each patient has a pressing need and it appears to be an almost impossible situation. How do you act in these patients' best interests?

Unfortunately, again, there are no easy answers as there are obviously risks attached to each patient. One thing that might be established is whether anyone else could help for a short period to overcome these difficulties. If this is the case, a possible solution might be to get another member of staff to look after the confused patient while you could quickly ensure that the patient who has the continence problem is placed on a clean sheet and has a continence pad in place until you have an opportunity to deal with the problem more thoroughly. You could then address the issue of preparing the patient for the invasive procedure. This is by no means a perfect solution – nurses are always having to make compromises and this type of situation does make nurses feel guilty that they cannot carry out caring activities effectively. Fullbrook (2008: 456) has identified this extremely well in highlighting that: 'bluntly, nurses have to be able to apply the principles to practice in such a way that reinforces their belief that they have succeeded in meeting their duty of clinical care'.

This is precisely the kind of scenario that unresolved staff shortages present nurses with. Not only does it have moral and ethical implications but should anything disastrous arise from these occurrences, there could be legal issues arising from same.

Obviously, the nurse in charge of the ward in the above scenario needs to make this dangerous situation known to the relevant manager; such a person has a responsibility to act on such information. It is a good idea for that nurse in charge to document the events and what action she or he took to resolve the situation and what help, if any, was given. The record should be signed and dated (in most trusts this would most likely be documented on an incident form) but a copy should be available somewhere should any incident, complaint, investigation or even evidence be required in a court of law at a later date. There is often a time lag in calling for such evidence and it is very difficult to remember dates, events, and so on much later.

Ethical decisions within the team

Sometimes moral decisions that others make are acceptable to you, and sometimes they are not. As nurses and midwives you work as part of a team and it can be difficult to gain a consensus about ethical issues. Consider the scenario in Exercise 6.4.

Exercise 6.4

You have a gentleman on your placement in a rehabilitation unit. Originally, this gentleman was admitted for rehabilitation following a stroke. He has become increasingly withdrawn and unco-operative and is refusing to eat. He is extremely frail, and the multiprofessional team are concerned about his health status. The registered nurse is concerned about this situation and decides to talk to his daughter who visits daily. During the discussion, the daughter says she thinks he may be missing his wife who is in a different hospital in the city receiving end-of-life care.

The nurse discusses this with the multiprofessional team and it is decided to try to get his wife into the rehabilitation unit to try and make this gentleman happy but also so that this couple can spend some time together.

The transfer of this gentleman's wife is fairly urgent as she is in the terminal stages of her illness. Unfortunately, the rehabilitation unit has a waiting list of eight patients waiting to come to the unit from the local acute hospital. However, most of the team agree to put this gentleman's wife at the top of the transfer list and organize this with the team looking after the gentleman's wife. One nurse within the team finds she doesn't necessarily agree with this decision as the unit is a rehabilitation unit and other patients may suffer because their rehabilitation is delayed. There are specific criteria that need to be met for admission to the rehabilitation unit and this decision would be breaking the rules as this lady does

> not fit the admission criteria. She also says that, in addition, other acutely ill patients in the acute hospital may suffer as in-patient beds are being taken up by patients awaiting a rehabilitation place at the unit.
>
> What would your view be of this decision by the multiprofessional team?

This is an interesting scenario to contemplate. Resources within a health care system can be scarce at times, and difficult decisions have to be made that may not be acceptable to the whole of the team. However, care and compassion should be at the heart of health care delivery, and the team's decision is a compassionate one. Sometimes rules may be broken in order to provide the best for the individuals concerned. However, before you disregard rules, it is important to remember that you will be accountable for the decisions you make and will be required to justify the decisions you make.

Legal issues in nursing

The issue of accountability was introduced briefly in Chapter 1, together with the fact that the nurse is accountable to the law, the professional body, the public and society. It was briefly discussed how, in terms of accountability, you have to be able to justify your decisions as you can be held to account for the decisions you make. Legally, you have to achieve the standards set out in the Code (NMC, 2008). The Code requires you to:

- respect your patients/clients as individuals
- you need to obtain consent before you give any treatment or care
- you have to maintain your patients'/clients' confidentiality
- you need to work collaboratively with team members
- you have to maintain your professional knowledge and competence, acknowledging your limitations in terms of competence
- you need to be trustworthy
- you need to act and identify risks to patients/clients, taking steps to minimize risks.

While it is not the remit of this chapter to address legal issues in depth, some common legal aspects are addressed within this section. Issues pertaining to consent, duty of care and documentation of care are explored using scenarios to highlight how you might cope with these issues in terms of decision making.

It should also be noted that often legal issues have ethical components as well as the fact that ethical issues often involve legal aspects of care.

Consent to treatment and care

Consent involves the patient/client being reasonably informed. Consent can often be implied by the patient, for example, if you ask a patient if it is okay to take his blood pressure and he rolls his sleeve up, and offers you his arm. This patient has not said anything but implies consent by his actions.

Express consent is often oral or written. For example, in the situation regarding blood pressure, the patient says 'Yes, it is fine to take my blood pressure.'

Written consent is usually asked for in situations where procedures are particularly invasive or carry high risks. When giving consent, the patient/client has a right to expect that the person undertaking the procedure is qualified and competent to carry out the procedure and the practitioner should ensure that consent is:

- freely given
- reasonably informed
- full.

For example, a person can refuse to take their medication. In terms of consent being freely given, it is still acceptable for the nurse to try and persuade a patient to take their tablets, but it is not acceptable for them to try and force a person to take tablets.

Being reasonably informed

Being reasonably informed involves explaining to a person what the care or treatment will involve, as well as the likely risks. However, too much information may frighten the person involved so much that they are too frightened to consent. Some years ago I nursed an elderly patient who had an inguinal hernia repaired. Twenty-four hours later, the patient bled profusely from the wound post-operatively. It was decided to take the patient back to theatre. The junior doctor who was to assist at the operation told the patient what they intended to do, what the general risks were, but also added that, of course, the patient may not wake up again from the anaesthetic as they had already had a general anaesthetic recently! This patient was then very frightened and shaking so much that when he tried to sign the consent form, he could not sign his name. Fortunately, his daughter was present. She ascertained verbally that her father wanted to consent to the surgery, and she signed the consent form for the patient as the next of kin. A complaint was subsequently received from the daughter about the information that had been given prior to the second operation.

Consider the scenario in Exercise 6.5.

Exercise 6.5

You are looking after Fred Jones, aged 85, who has been admitted to your ward for abdominal surgery, which will result in the formation of a permanent stoma. Fred has signed a consent form but tells you that he does not really understand the procedure to be carried out as the doctor was called to an emergency and left before being able to give full details of the operation. The doctor has not returned since.

- What are the ethical and legal issues that arise from this scenario?
- What decisions would you make to try and remedy this situation?

Consent

The issue here lies around 'consent'. The patient has admitted to not understanding what he has signed for – he might well have been given an explanation by the doctor but it is quite probable that his understanding was not checked by the doctor obtaining the consent, in view of the emergency that interrupted this procedure.

Ritchie and Reynard (2008: 48) in an editorial concerning consent have called for a standardized NHS consent checklist to overcome the potential problem of inadequate consenting procedures. They assert that: 'A surgeon who fails to consent a patient adequately for an operation is in breach of [the] duty of care to that patient.'

The problem posed for the nurse in this example is a possible time lag in allaying the patient's anxieties and how much information should a nurse give to the patient in this instance?

Again, Ritchie and Reynard (2008) have posed the issue about how much information should be given about surgical procedures while minimizing anxieties. For this reason, a standardized checklist that may include images, diagrams and generic complications may help. Too much information on everything that can possibly go wrong can mean that a person will withhold their consent as they are then too frightened to agree to a procedure.

It is obviously vital that a nurse must know his or her patient well to be able to judge accurately what that particular patient needs in the way of information in order to be able to understand what that patient has consented to.

Again, difficulties are posed in the way of currently admitting patients only shortly before a (non-emergency) surgical procedure takes place. In those circumstances, any pre-operative assessment must include information about the procedures, what risks are involved, and a check on the patient's understanding.

Jolley (2007: 39) has reinforced this by stating that: 'staff have an ethical duty to provide information about any interventions'.

Booth (2002), in a discussion relating to informed consent, identified some patients' hesitancy in asking medical staff for further information/clarification. This often puts nurses in a difficult position when faced by a patient who does not understand what they might have signed up to. It is often a problem presented to student nurse – how do they select the right decision in this case?

As to the decision you make in the circumstances, you need to seek advice. The ideal would be for the doctor to return to deal with the situation but this could take time and Mr Jones could become more and more anxious. It might therefore be appropriate for a qualified member of the nursing staff to advise Mr Jones and answer his questions. It would be valuable for the student to be present when this happens, so if something similar occurred in the same area, you would be aware of how to deal with it. (This equates with the second stage of the 'add on framework' for decision making – taking into account peer/expert opinion and clinical experience contributing to future decisions.)

Exercise 6.6

You are looking after Steve, a 19-year-old type 1 diabetic. He has been admitted to your medical ward as a result of him being found in a state of depressed consciousness and was subsequently diagnosed as being in a ketotic state. He has been stabilized on the ward and the consultant physician has asked him to remain on the ward for a further two days in order that the diabetic specialist nurse can see him to give him help and education about his disorder. After the medical staff have left, he calls you and tells you that he has no intention of staying any longer in the hospital and wants to discharge himself.

- What are the ethical and legal issues that arise from this scenario?
- What decisions would you make to try and remedy this situation?

Duty of care

This is where the issue of duty of care arises. You want to act in the patient's best interests but unless that patient is detained under a section of the Mental Health Act, the patient cannot be forced to remain in the area. This is both an ethical and a legal problem. Nurses have a duty of care towards the patients for whom they are responsible and accountable but the dilemma occurs when a patient refuses to cooperate.

The first step would be to try and find out why he does not want to stay in your unit. There may be something that can be relatively easily dealt with such as a problem at home, or there may be some event that has occurred on the ward during his stay that has precipitated this reaction.

Failing to identify something that can easily be dealt with, a senior nurse needs to be involved with this patient (at least you then have a witness). With a witness you can try and persuade the patient to stay, explaining why and how it will benefit him. The senior nurse may also be aware of factors affecting this individual that you are unaware of that she can rectify.

If these actions fail to persuade the patient, it would be useful to get a member of the medical staff to return as soon as possible to deal with the situation.

This is a situation where documentation is of vital importance, and documenting details of the situation should occur as near to the event as possible. In the event of some untoward event should the patient insist on leaving without completing his treatment, you will at least have the evidence of the steps you took, and in which order.

The scope of your duty of care covers everything you do in relation to a patient, including negligence through an act or omission on your part. You have a legal obligation to ensure that any act or omission on your part does not cause harm to your patient. We have already explored within this chapter how difficult that can be at times. However, should any legal issue arise from the care that you deliver, the whole situation would be taken into account. This is why it is important to document events as well as the rationales for your decisions. You need to be very clear why you chose a particular course of action so that you can more readily justify your decisions to others. In addition, as a student, you should consult more experienced staff especially your mentor. Part of the mentoring process is to learn from the experience of others.

You should also bear in mind that the scope of your duty of care encompasses:

- the care given to a patient
- giving advice
- explaining risks and procedures
- documenting legibly in nursing notes and when giving instructions
- maintaining good standards of record-keeping
- the timing of your decision to act
- seeking the assistance of others
- only acting within your sphere of competence
- ensuring you do not fail to report substandard care if you observe this.

Source: Griffith and Tengnah (2008).

The last point made can be extremely difficult for a student to cope with. The RCN (2004) give guidance on whistle-blowing identifying that all workers are protected under the Public Interest Disclosure Act 1998. The guidance states that the term 'workers' includes students. The RCN highlights that under the Act you are required to have a reasonable belief that your information is correct when reporting situations and that you need to raise the issue internally to a responsible person (this could include a legal adviser) and feel it is appropriate to disclose the information to the person you are reporting any issue to. The area in which you are working may have a whistle-blowing procedure that you might be able to consult. In addition, there are other resources that you can use for advice such as the NMC Professional Advice service.

Consider Exercise 6.7 to enable you to think about how you might proceed if you observed substandard care.

Exercise 6.7

You are working with a health care assistant who is very conscientious about completing tasks for patients. However, you notice that she is extremely abrupt with patients, and fails to pick up on their non-verbal cues such as whether they are in pain.

You find a patient in tears after she has helped this patient to have a wash and get out of bed into a chair. The patient tells you that the care assistant was very rough with her, even though she had tried to tell her she needed some painkillers before she could face having a wash.

You are upset about this and say you will ask the staff nurse to get her some painkillers straight away. The patient thanks you but then says please don't tell anyone about the care assistant as she doesn't want to get anyone into trouble.

Consider the courses of action available to you and list these. Which course of action do you think would be most appropriate here in terms of maintaining your duty of care to this patient?

You could do as the patient asks and do nothing. However, you would be failing in your duty of care to the patient. Another course of action might be to explain to the patient that you will need to speak to the care assistant and explain the outcomes of her actions, asking her to be more considerate of the patients' needs. However, this could be quite daunting for you as a second-year nurse and, of course, may have no impact on this individual's behaviour. As a second-year student, it would probably be most appropriate to highlight this issue with your mentor. The mentor will then be able to follow this up with the care assistant concerned, and may even need to speak to the placement manager about this. You will, however, need to document what you observed and what the patient said to you. You must be careful how you do this and only document facts, not how you have interpreted them. Documentation requirements will be dealt with in more detail later in the next section. The essential requirement here is to fulfil your duty of care to the patient to protect this patient from any further harm.

Exercise 6.8 Child branch

You are allocated to care for Bethany aged 16 who has an eating disorder, anorexia nervosa. She has been referred to tier 4 of Community and Mental Health Services (CAMHS) services; however, there is currently no in-patient bed available and as an interim measure she has been admitted to the paediatric medical ward. Bethany has become increasingly agitated since admission and is currently refusing all food, but is continuing to drink copious amounts of water. Her parents have encouraged staff to undertake whatever measures are deemed necessary.

● What are the legal and ethical issues that arise from this scenario?
● What decisions would you make to try and remedy this situation?

A young person aged 16 does have a statutory right to consent to treatment under the provisions of the Family Law Reform Act (1969). However, just because Bethany is aged over 16, this does not mean that she is competent to consent. Bethany's case would need to be considered under the Mental Capacity Act (2005) since this does apply to young people aged 16 years and over and there is evidence to suggest that she is not competent to make a decision. Anorexia nervosa is recognized to be an illness that does affect the ability of the young person to make an informed decision. In this situation consideration has to be given to Bethany's best interests. The refusal of treatment can be overridden by Bethany's parents (those with parental responsibility) or by a court order when it is considered to be in her best interests. In this situation it could be argued that by continuing to refuse food this could result in either permanent damage/disability or even death. Therefore, the rights of young people aged 16–18 can be overridden to preserve their long-term interests and they do not have the same legal status to consent and refuse treatment as adults.

Clearly, in this situation, it would be beneficial if the situation can be resolved without the courts becoming involved. In the first instance you do need to advise either your mentor and/or the senior nurse in charge of the situation. It would be beneficial to try and get the paediatric consultant to become involved and discuss with Bethany as to why she has been admitted and the consequences of her refusing to eat to see if her co-operation can be secured. You would need to ascertain whether Bethany wants her parents to be involved in these discussions; however, she does need to be aware that they will be kept appraised of what is happening and being discussed. Maintaining effective communication with Bethany, her parents and all health and social care professionals involved is essential. This is a situation where accurate documentation is essential and you will need to keep comprehensive records of action taken and advice given. You may be required to account for your actions and advice.

Consideration also needs to be given as to whether the paediatric ward is an appropriate environment for Bethany to be cared for. Access to emergency CAMHS may need to be further investigated. In addition, it may be necessary to consider whether as a student you are equipped with the knowledge and skills required to care for this young person. It may be more appropriate for a qualified nurse to be allocated to care for Bethany and for you to be involved as appropriate. Additionally, thought should be given as to whether there is a risk that Bethany may harm herself and whether she should be constantly observed in order to ensure that she is kept safe.

Documentation

Another issue that certainly has legal implications is the issue of documentation and whether the documentation is written or electronic. This is a crucial element in the nurses' role as documentation is required to give an account of the patient's care and treatment; it helps in monitoring a person's progress, and communicates information to other staff. Patient records can also be required as evidence should there be a complaint or legal issue arise, and it is therefore important to make a record of care, events or incidents as soon as possible after contact with a patient/client. In addition to these elements, it is important to document decisions about care giving some detail as to how your decisions have been reached (Griffith and Tengnah, 2008).

It can be difficult to know how much detail to record at times. As a student, you need to have entries in patient records countersigned by a registered nurse/midwife. This is useful in learning how much detail to include as you can discuss this aspect with your mentor. Records should be able to be read by another person who will then have a clear picture of what you have experienced.

Your records need to be legible, clear and unambiguous, free from abbreviations, accurate, impartial and chronological. While in placement areas, you may observe staff undertaking an audit of records and the Audit Commission (2002) state that this is the best way to ensure high-quality record-keeping.

Handing information over to other staff

Handing over information to other staff is a vital component of the nurse/midwives role.

Exercise 6.9

Think about the last time you had to document your patient's care and give handover to other staff. How did you decide which information was relevant to include in your documentation and handover?

Documenting care and preparing to hand over patients to other staff require decisions to be made about what needs to be documented/handed over. Include all details of what has occurred will impact on time management and may result in staff losing the impetus to read or listen to your account. Hence, you need to be current, concise and informative about the patient's current status in order to provide other staff/ professionals with enough information to be able to continue care in a seamless manner. What you include involves an element of judgement. Discussing with your mentor prior to completing documentation or giving handover to other staff what you intend to include is a useful exercise in ensuring you include all relevant information. It is also useful to discuss with your mentor after completion of these aspects of care to ask for feedback on your performance/documentation skills.

Patient handover to other staff depends on accurate record-keeping, with records being the basis of what you hand over to others.

Exercise 6.10

Think back over the handovers you have received from staff. What sort of elements does a handover have to contain?

When giving, or receiving handover from other staff, it is important to ensure:

- information is correct
- it gives you a clear understanding of the person's problems and diagnosis
- you receive current information about the individual that includes all relevant aspects of that person's situation
- the information is concise
- the handover enables you to know what has been done for that person, you know about any referrals made, and you are aware of what still needs to be done.

Ideally, a handover should also give you the opportunity to ask questions about that person and anything you are unclear about. However, many handover styles today mean it is difficult to clarify information during this process. For example, many placement areas tape their handover of patients or construct a printed handover sheet, rather than talking face to face. While these methods do appear to minimize the time spent on handover, they make it difficult to ask questions and use the handover as a learning exercise. This is particularly apparent for novice students. To overcome this, it is useful to carry a notebook in your pocket so you can jot down any issues that require clarification for you. You can then ask your mentor or another member of staff these questions at a convenient time during your span of duty.

Consider the scenario in Exercise 6.11 that highlights the importance of good documenting skills.

Exercise 6.11 Mental health

You are working in a ward that cares for elderly patients who have mental health problems and dementia. One of the patients, Mr Thomas, has been admitted to the ward having been transferred from another hospital. Mr Thomas is unable to give a history of events so you and your mentor are reliant on the transfer documentation to enable you to care for this patient. There is very little information given about the patient apart from his dementia state. Mr Thomas has been commenced upon a regime of tricyclic antidepressants before his transfer. You measure his vital signs and find that his pulse is very slow and irregular. There is no mention in the medical or nursing transfer notes of cardiac disease. It is a known fact that tricyclic antidepressants can make cardiac problems worse.

What legal issues might have followed from this if this matter had not been discovered?

This situation illustrates the necessity to document care very carefully. Documentation forms a vital link in the chain of communication. What might have followed from this incident had the problem not been identified could have had serious implications for this patient. A cardiac emergency could have been precipitated resulting in the death of the patient. This situation would have been investigated in both the transferring and receiving hospitals. It would most likely have been the subject of a coroner's enquiry. In such a situation the documentation would have been scrutinized very carefully and blame apportioned to the parties who had omitted to document relevant facts. You need to note that documentation needs to be 'contemporaneous'. This means that records need to be completed immediately after events occur. If documentation is completed after too long a period, it is difficult to remember events correctly.

Conclusion

You should have realized from working through these scenarios how ethics and legal issues affect nursing care. You will also begin to incorporate Stage 2 of the 'add on framework' for decision making. When dealing with such events as described in the above case study scenarios, you will certainly require the opinion of your peers and from experts in your current clinical situations. When reflecting on such incidents, try to access teaching staff in your higher education establishments who have experience in this field as you will find it helpful for future similar events.

In addition, reflecting on situations, identifying what your learning needs are, following this up by identifying ways in which you can meet those learning needs, and following this through until you have met those learning needs will add to the repertoire of skills and knowledge that you accumulate that will be of benefit in future situations.

References

Audit Commission (2002) *Setting the Record Straight*. London: Audit Commission.

Beauchamp, T.L. and Childress, J.F. (1989) *Principles of Biomedical Ethics*, 3rd edn. Oxford: Oxford University Press.

Booth, S. (2002) A philosophical analysis of informed consent, *Nursing Standard*, 16(39): 43–6.

Fullbrook, S. (2007) Best interests: a review of issues that affect nurses' decision making, *British Journal of Nursing*, 16(10): 600–1.

Fullbrook, S. (2008) Duty of care and political expectations (Part 2: Readers' concerns/experiences), *British Journal of Nursing*, 17(7): 456–7.

Griffith, R. and Tengnah, C. (2008) *Law and Professional Issues in Nursing*. Exeter: Learning Matters Ltd.

Jolley, S. (2007) An audit of patients' understanding of routine pre-operative investigations, *Nursing Standard*, 21(22): 35–9.

Llewellyn, A. and Hayes, S. (2008) *Fundamentals of Nursing Care*. Exeter: Reflect Press Ltd.

Nursing and Midwifery Council (NMC) (2008) *The Code: Standards of Conduct, Performance and Ethics for Nurses and Midwives*. London: NMC.

Nursing and Midwifery Council (NMC) (2009) *Guidance for the Care of Older People*. London: NMC.

Nursing and Midwifery Council (NMC) *Professional Advice Service*, available online at www.nmc-org.uk.

Ritchie, R. and Reynard, J. (2008) Consent for surgery: time for a standardized NHS consent checklist, *Journal of the Royal Society of Medicine*, 101(2): 48–9.

Royal College of Nursing (RCN) (2004) *Blowing the Whistle*. London: RCN.

Thiroux, J. and Krasemann, K. (2007) *Ethics, Theory and Practice*, 9th edn. Upper Saddle River, NJ, Pearson and Prentice Hall.

Tschudin, V. (2003) *Ethics in Nursing*, 3rd edn. Edinburgh: Butterworth Heinemann.

Vestal, R. (2008) Managing interruptions, *Nurse Leader*, 6(3): 8–9.

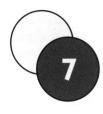

7 Increasing complexity in decision making

- **Introduction**
- **Managing care**
- **Handing over patient information**
- **Talking to patients**
- **Planning and time management**
- **Managing a small group of patients – prioritizing care**
- **Time and resource allocation**
- **Delegation**
- **Time management**
- **Asking for help**
- **Adapting plans**
- **Factors that can enhance or constrain decision making**
- **Conclusion**
- **References**

Introduction

In Chapter 6 we introduced some legal and ethical factors that can influence decision-making, and started to introduce your developing role as a more senior student. We also explored individual decisions made by the nurse/midwife. However, as you progress through your course you need to expand these skills into looking after a small group of patients. Decision making becomes more complex when managing a group of patients and often requires you to 'think on your feet' and respond quickly. This means you need to start out with a structure/framework for that group of patients in order to try and use your resources effectively.

Managing care

By the time you are managing care for groups of patients, you should be working to Bondy Level 4. This level requires you to practise proficiently, with your mentor acting as your point of reference if you are unsure of how to proceed. Your actions should be underpinned with sound evidence-based rationales that reflect decision making Stage 3 in the framework outlined in Chapter 1. In addition, when managing care, you should demonstrate your ability to adapt your behaviour/interventions to the needs of your clients and the environment of care.

Exercise 7.1

List the resources available to you when managing a group of patients.

You may have thought of:

- your experience and knowledge
- your mentor
- other staff
- physical resources such as enough bed linen
- time.

Managing a group of patients requires you to think about making decisions about:

- how you utilize information that has been handed over to you by previous staff
- deciding if you need more information
- assessing or reassessing patients
- prioritizing care
- planning care
- deciding what to delegate and who you can delegate to
- how to manage your time effectively
- how to respond to changes/incidents/issues that arise
- adapting your initial plans.

At first glance this appears to be a daunting task. In your first few placements this would have been impossible to achieve. You need to draw on your previous nursing experience; remember your mentors and how they coped with this, and use the knowledge/evidence you have acquired. It will seem a daunting task but, with practice, discussion with your mentor and through reflection on experiences, you will start to develop management skills until they occur in a fluent and rapid manner. Like all skills, you need to practise in order to become proficient.

Exercise 7.2

Think about what you do at the start of a span of duty. Before you start to look after patients, what is it necessary to do?

The first thing you do is find out about the patients you are going to be looking after. This may take the form of handover from previous staff or reading the patients' documentation.

Handing over patient information

Ideally, a handover should also give you the opportunity to ask questions about that person and anything you are unclear about.

See pp. 103–4 for a list of the important elements of a handover. However, at intershift handover, with the best intentions, the handover cannot give you a complete picture about a patient. There are other sources of information that will help you gain a complete picture about patient care.

Talking to patients

In addition to taking a handover, you need to talk to the patients you are going to be managing, or their relatives/carers. These sources are invaluable in terms of helping you to understand the complete picture about a person.

If the patients are in a location together, it is also helpful when walking into that environment to visually scan the patients. This allows you to pick up on non-verbal cues from patients and helps you to decide who you need to go to first. Making these sorts of observation helps towards prioritizing patient needs.

Looking at the individual's nursing documentation, including any observation charts, measurement charts, and prescription charts will also add useful information as to the person's current status, and what you might be required to do for them. If other health care professionals are involved with a particular individual, it is useful to consult their notes also. This is especially important if you do not have multiprofessional notes within the placement.

Planning and time management

Planning care is about deciding what care needs to be delivered. Planning is necessary in order to maximize your time and to use other resources available to you more effectively. Effective planning and time management are a good foundation for delivering effective patient care. Without effective planning, care can be disorganized with elements being forgotten or the nurse running out of time to complete essential care. There is a close relationship between time management and stress, and managing time appropriately is a way to reduce stress and increase productivity (Marquis and Huston, 2009). In addition, the decisions you make when planning your shift can impact on other health care professionals who are also endeavouring to deliver effective care to patients.

It would be good to work within an environment where there were more than adequate resources to be able to achieve everything you would wish for your patients. However, the reality is that you often need to make decisions about what you can achieve within a given period of time and make compromises that will not put your patients at risk in any way. This can be difficult at times. This is reflected in Price's (2008) writing that the nurse faces compromises between individualizing nursing care and meeting centrally set targets. He also goes on to say that sometimes the professional ethos taught in the university can be difficult to practise given the constraints placed on health care delivery. This is why reflective discussions with your mentor, peers and personal reflections can benefit you by learning from your experience, helping to guide you towards safe compromises. Reflecting with others is particularly useful as they may reveal different insights into the decisions they might have made. This is not to say that your decisions were necessarily incorrect. There may not be any clear-cut answers in some situations you deal with. However, reflective discussions can expand your views, insights and rationales for decisions reached that may be useful in the future, or which may help you to enhance your decision making skills should you face similar situations in the future.

Managing a small group of patients – prioritizing care

Try the example in Exercise 7.3 to consider options available when managing patient care.

Exercise 7.3

You are working in an asthma clinic. You have three patients in the waiting room who are waiting to be seen.

Patient 1 on the list: attending for a routine check-up and review of medication. The patient is sitting reading a book.

Patient 2 on the list: a follow-up appointment after a hospital admission for an exacerbation of his asthma. This patient is looking at his watch and seems a little agitated.

Patient 3 on the list: due for a review of medication. Is extremely breathless, coughing a lot, looks very flushed and is leaning forward onto another chair for support.

 What choices are available to you in this situation?

 What are the potential consequences for each option available to you?

Option 1: you can choose to call the patients to see the doctor in the order they are booked in for. If you do this though, patient 3 remains distressed and the patient's condition may deteriorate further.

Option 2: you could ask the doctor to see patient 3 first as the patient appears to be in some respiratory distress. This may result in the other two becoming annoyed because they are kept waiting.

Option 3: you can ask the doctor to see patient 3 first but go straight back to explain the reasons for your choice and that the doctor will resume the correct order as soon as he has dealt with patient 3. This option addresses not only the apparent emergency but also addresses essential communication skills. If patients are given reasons and some reassurance about time-scales, they are less likely to complain. Remember, they do not always appreciate the reasons they are kept waiting even if the rationales for decisions are readily apparent to yourself.

Prioritizing care is important in order to prevent further emergencies occurring and in order to maximize your time management. A simple scheme for helping you to prioritize care has been suggested as:

A   Must be done
B   Should be done
C   Could be done

Source: Adapted from Siviter (2008).

So, how can Siviter's scheme be applied in practice? Consider the following scenario.

It is 8.00 a.m. and you have been allocated three patients to look after.

Patient A: this patient is due to go to theatre at 9 a.m. and needs to be prepared promptly.

Patient B: this patient has to remain on bedrest and is demanding to have a wash. She says he has been asking for a wash since before the night staff went off duty. This lady also says she wants her hair washed before she attends to her hygiene needs.

Patient C: this lady is in severe pain and is asking for some pain relief. She also wants the telephone to call her sister to ask her if she will bring in some fresh night-clothes.

Using Siviter's scheme, the following might be decided:

- *Must*: the pain relief for patient C is a priority and you need to ask your mentor to supervise you in this. The second priority is to get patient A ready for theatre as, if you do not, this impacts on the theatre list and will impact on the work of the theatre porters in collecting patients for theatre.

- *Should*: you should help patient B to have a wash as soon as possible. However, if you explain why the patient has to wait a short while and indicate the approximate time you can get to the patient, this will help to reassure patient B that you have not forgotten them.

- *Could*: it will probably make this patient feel more comfortable if they have their hair washed but you may have to explain why this may have to wait until later in the day. In addition, you will probably have to explain to patient C that you will get the telephone as soon as you have completed other tasks, or you could ask if the ward clerk could make the call for patient C.

Deciding on patient priorities can be difficult. It is not always easy to please all patients/clients immediately. However, in communicating why things cannot be done straight away, by giving some thought to your dilemma and giving information about when you might be able to meet a person's needs, this can reduce anxiety for your patients/clients and, in doing so, reduce your own stress.

Try the example in Exercise 7.4 to practise setting priorities when managing care.

Exercise 7.4   Mental health nursing

Peter Hathaway is a 20-year-old undergraduate student at the local university. He has had recurrent periods of depression since the death of his girlfriend in a road traffic accident a year earlier in which he was the driver. Peter has been supported by his general practitioner but, unfortunately, Peter's periods of depression are becoming longer in duration and of greater depth. His friends report that he spends a great deal of his time alone in his room, will not socialize, and just keeps on repeating that he wants to be with his girlfriend. As the examination period of the university approaches, Peter isolates himself in his room and becomes even more withdrawn. He does not respond to any contact and after five days, he is found severely dehydrated and malnourished. His personal hygiene is poor and it is apparent that he has remained bedridden during this period and has urinated and defecated in the bed. He expresses a monosyllabic poverty of speech and his movements are profoundly retarded.

   He is admitted to the acute Mental Health In-Patient Services of your local hospital.

   At the time of Peter's admission what would be the immediate priorities of care?

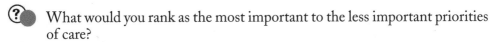

What would you rank as the most important to the less important priorities of care?

What are your reasons for these decisions?

Now consider the priorities of care for the first 72 hours.

What would you consider priorities of care within this first 72 hours? Again, consider how you would rank the priorities from those that are most important to those that are less important.

What factors did you take into account in prioritizing these care needs? How do they differ from the initial priorities of care above?

Note: You will need to think about whether you will address physical or emotional needs first for each part of the scenario. It may also be useful to think about when Peter is going to be at most risk of self-harm.

You may now wish to use some examples from your portfolio, or one of the following exercises to continue to practise establishing priorities of care for patients.

Exercise 7.5

Community nursing

You are accompanying the district nurse to visit a gentleman who lives alone. He has reduced mobility, and can only manage to get around the house using a walking aid. He has recently experienced occasions of urinary incontinence and the district nurse wants to supervise you undertaking an assessment of this gentleman. You knock at the door but there is no answer. You are a little concerned as this is quite unusual for this gentleman. You try to check with the neighbours if he is all right. However, the neighbours are out. You call his next of kin on your mobile phone but they say he was not planning to go out. They live some distance away and do not have access to the property.

What will your priorities be in this situation?

What options are available to you?

Which option will you choose, giving your reasons for your decision?

Day centre care

Attending the day centre is a service user who has challenging behaviour. He has become very aggressive and unco-operative in the presence of other service users who are attending a painting class. He is lashing out physically at another service user whom he has become quite agitated with before.

 What are your immediate priorities here, and why?

 Once you have sorted out this immediate situation, how will your priorities change in relation to this service user?

 Explain the reasons for your subsequent decisions.

Time and resource allocation

Along with prioritizing comes the issue of time allocation. This is possibly one of the most difficult aspects of nursing work to cope with.

It can be difficult to plan your time allocation as there are many things that can impact on the decisions that you have made in terms of priorities. You can start a span of duty organizing your priorities for the individuals allocated to you but it can be difficult to estimate how much time you need for each individual task. For example, you may estimate that it might take you 30 minutes to wash a patient. However, while washing the patient they may become upset that necessitates you finding out about the cause of the person's distress. This may take additional time that you have not catered for in your plan but becomes a priority in that particular instance. This means that you have to 'think on your feet' in terms of resetting your priorities and allocating time to other tasks.

You will probably be surprised at all the elements that can affect the nurse's use of time. In addition to the needs of your patients/clients, there may be many interruptions to your original plan. These may include:

- unexpected demands on your time, for example, an unplanned discharge or admission of a patient
- unexpected incidents occurring, for example, a patient falling out of bed
- demands from other health care professionals such as the medical staff wanting to undertake an unplanned ward round
- telephone calls from other departments or patients' relatives that require you to act on aspects of care
- other staff asking for assistance with their patients/clients.

The subject of time management for nurses does not appear to have been studied extensively but some studies have shown that exhortation to nurses to use time effectively have sometimes resulted in stress, burnout and a feeling of guilt due to not always being able to deliver patient care as one would wish (Waterworth et al., 1999;

Bowers et al., 2001; Kalisch et al., 2009). As previously discussed, the stress experienced may not be through a lack of planning by yourself, but due to unexpected circumstances beyond your control.

This is why we discussed the legal, professional and ethical issues in Chapter 6 that can impact on you when making decisions, particularly when staff and other resources are scarce. This has also been identified in the USA by Volker (2003: 210) when: 'healthcare professionals experience organisational and interdisciplinary ethical conflicts that arise from practising in environments fraught with shrinking resources and conflicting values'.

This is why it is so important to consider planning and time management together.

Delegation

We have to prioritize when we are caring for groups of patients and delegation is a key skill you will need to develop when managing care in order to cope with the variety of situations that can arise. What you are able to delegate will very much depend on the outcome of your patient assessment and the skills and experience that the care assistant has. It is important you are aware of his or her abilities and competence as you will remain responsible and accountable for the tasks you decide to delegate. The issues surrounding delegation of tasks to support workers are highlighted within nursing literature (Hansten and Washburn, 1996; Boucher, 1998; Simon, 1998; RCN, 2006). In particular, Boucher (1998) raises the issue of support workers being trained to undertake tasks but not trained in critical thinking, which would require them to interpret cues. This then means that, in your role as delegator, you need to be explicit in what the support worker needs to do, what he or she needs to look for in the patient and what they should report to you. Therefore, effective communication is a fundamental element of delegation. The RCN (2006) sets out key principles to guide practitioners when delegating, as does the NMC (2008) stating:

- You must establish that anyone you delegate to is able to carry out your instructions.
- You must confirm the outcome of any delegated task meets the required standards.
- You must make sure that everyone you are responsible for is supervised and supported.

In addition, you will need to liaise with your mentor in terms of what you are delegating as he or she will also be delegating tasks to the care assistant. You must try to ensure that, in delegating, you do not overload the person you are delegating to, causing them stress and distress.

Exercise 7.6

Reflect on the times that you have had tasks delegated to you. Think about how the delegation was done.

How did it make you feel?

 Was the delegation appropriate?

 If not, why not?

As indicated previously, you will still be under the supervision of a qualified nurse/ midwife but as you progress through your final clinical placements as a student, you will be expected to develop the skill of delegating to others. This is obviously a daunting task. While it might seem easier for you to delegate to a junior nursing/midwifery student, how do you cope with an experienced health care assistant? This care assistant may have worked in the clinical setting for a number of years, knows the routines and the type of patient cared for and will probably have done some study (mandatory and other). How will they feel about you delegating work to them? There may well be other parties to whom you need to delegate (possibly lay carers, relatives and other support workers in the area – ward clerks, for example). In considering this topic, what actually is delegation? The NMC (2008: 3) specify that it is: 'The transfer to a competent individual the authority to perform a specified situation that can be carried out in the absence of that nurse or midwife and without direct supervision.'

Whatever you decide to delegate (and whoever you decide to delegate to), it must be in the best interests of the patient. It must also be a suitable task to delegate; the person undertaking the delegated task must be competent and must be willing (considering their own capability) to accept the request. This requires very careful judgement. Consider the situation in Exercise 7.7.

Exercise 7.7

You are in your final placement as a student nurse on a general medical ward. You have been allocated a bay of patients (6) for the shift and a health care assistant who has been working in the area for six months is available to you. One patient needs his vital signs checking on an hourly basis and in this area, these are done by means of a machine. You decide to ask the health care assistant to do this for you as you have other pressing matters to attend to at this point.

How would you approach her to undertake this task and what does she need to know in order to carry it out safely?

The first question is, would you actually delegate it or do the task yourself? You may feel that due to the equipment used and the state of the patients that it may well be beyond the competence of this person. If, however, she states that she has done this before, what should you do?

You could observe her to satisfy yourself that she is able to perform this correctly or, you could demonstrate the skill and supervise her until you are happy that she is competent, reminding her that should there be any doubt as to her ability, she must make this known to you.

Delegation of care (if done properly) can be advantageous to both parties (delegator and delegate). For the delegator, it means that crucial other care work can be carried out on times, thus relieving stress and will be beneficial for the patients. For the delegate, it can bring job satisfaction, help with their development and give them a sense of worth. On the other hand, poor, ineffective delegation will be a disaster and will increase risks to patients. Do not forget that there are other support facilities that might be available to you. Ward clerks can often undertake tasks for nurses such as chasing results and notes, taking telephone calls – all of which can impinge on a nurse's time, taking him or her away from direct patient care.

Delegating to a student nurse/midwife might appear easier – the student will most likely be more junior to yourself and you will most likely have undertaken the same course and have an idea of the input that they have received from the educational institution. However, there is a note of caution. It could well be that the student has had a variety of placements and may not have practised all their clinical skills (or it could be their first clinical experience). You will need to satisfy yourself about their competence in order to undertake the task

---

Exercise 7.8

You are working in the same medical ward on a different shift. The area is very busy, two staff have reported sick and the trust has provided a health care assistant from a local agency to fill the gap.

How would you go about the task if you wanted to delegate vital signs measurements to this co-worker?

It should also have been made clear to you at the commencement of your clinical experience exactly what the health care assistants can and cannot do. However, in asking her politely could she help you by undertaking this task, you may need to ask her if she is happy using the machine. You also need to ask her to report the findings to you to keep you appraised of the situation. It is crucial that such measurements are carried out accurately – subsequent treatment will be based on such results – and if done incorrectly, it could pose a risk for the patient. Always remember to thank co-workers if they have carried out tasks for you; if you show respect to them, they may be more willing in times of crisis to help out at very short notice and 'pull out the stops' to resolve the situation.

Try the example in Exercise 7.9, or use the exercise guidelines to explore a span of duty in which you have cared for a group of patients and in which you had to delegate to others.

Exercise 7.9   Adult nursing

You are given three patients to manage care for a span of duty from 7 a.m. until 1 p.m. Your mentor says she will be available if you need help. The mentor has six other patients to manage. There is also a care assistant who is available to help you. The care assistant is supporting both you and your mentor.

Consider the patient profiles in Table 7.1 (*adult branch*)

❶ Describe the decisions you would make regarding nursing care for each patient in terms of priority, i.e. what must, should or could be done.
❷ What would you be able to delegate to the care assistant?

This exercise would be useful to include in your portfolio of learning.

Time management

In terms of being able to manage your time effectively, you need to consider a list of what needs to be done for each patient, estimating the amount of time care will take. From such a list, you can then begin to decide what must, could or should be done (Siviter, 2008). For example, nutritional needs are quite a high priority as is pain relief for these patients. In addition, Mr Saddiq's daughter needs some support and information about what will happen over the span of duty, and when. Another priority would be to inform Mr Brown's relatives of his change in condition, as well as the need to give medication to Mr Brown to ease his breathing and dry secretions on his chest.

You will also need to liaise with your mentor regarding medicine administration to ensure you do not impact on her prioritization for the needs of the patients she is caring for. Hygiene needs and observations (apart from Mr Saddiq's blood glucose monitoring) can be dealt with later. It may also take some planning to ensure that both you and the care assistant are together to help Mr Brown and Mr Wright with their hygiene needs. There are obviously other needs these patients have, and it is also important while delivering any care to ensure a kind, professional and emotionally supportive manner.

When managing a group of patients, the nurse/midwife also needs to ensure that meal breaks are planned for staff, while not forgetting to consider ward/placement routines that may impact on your decisions, for example, consultant ward rounds. Managing more than one patient while having to take into account the ward routine

Patient description	Planned and delegated care
Mr Wright is an 87-year-old man who is two weeks post-operative after having a hemicolectomy for cancer. He has a colostomy that he cannot deal with himself as he had a stroke six years ago. He can move all his limbs but has a severe tremor and is quite weak. His short-term memory is also not very good and he does get sudden periods when he is confused. He also has a skin condition that requires an application of emollient cream all over his body after washing. He has a poor appetite and needs encouragement to eat. He is still in some pain in his abdomen as he has a wound infection. He also has urgency to micturate and often cannot get to use his urinal in time	
Mr Saddiq is 82 years old and has been admitted for a refashioning of his colostomy. He has type 1 diabetes Mellitus, has a history of hypertension and mild heart failure. He requires insulin injections twice a day. He cannot speak much English, but his daughter is with him and acts as an interpreter. His daughter demands that you attend to her father's needs before going to anyone else	
Mr Brown had a laparotomy 10 days ago. It was found that he had inoperable cancer with metastases. He is in extreme pain from metastases in his spine. He is on the end of life care pathway. He has a son and daughter who live some distance away who don't visit often but keep informed via the telephone. Mr Brown is emaciated; he is aware but not able to communicate well. His breathing is quite laboured this morning and his chest gurgles. He is not eating at the moment and can only take sips of fluid with some encouragement	

Table 7.1   Managing patient care

and other health professionals' priorities can all seem extremely daunting, and this is why it is important to take time to assess the situation, make decisions about priorities and develop a plan. It is also the reason why you need to seek feedback from your mentor and reflect on how you manage any span of duty. We can all make errors in judgement when making decisions about the care we deliver. The important elements are to learn to recognize errors, learn from them, and develop action plans to work at enhancing our decision making ability. It is also useful to review current literature on a regular basis to learn about the theory of time management and prioritizing care. This will help you to reflect on your performance and can often inform the action plans you put in place for your future development.

Asking for help

You may feel that by asking for help in managing that you are admitting you are not very good, or failing in terms of management. This is not the case. If you feel out of your depth and do not know where to begin, it is important to recognize this and make the decision to seek advice. You are a supernumerary student who is in a placement to learn, and deciding when to seek help demonstrates you are recognizing your limitations but are willing to learn and develop.

Adapting plans

It is important to spend time assessing, planning, prioritizing and deciding what to delegate but you also need to recognize that you need to be adaptable and flexible with the plans you make should emergencies occur or situations change.

Exercise 7.10

While doing the medicine round with your mentor, your patient Mr Saddiq (see Table 7.1) collapses while walking to the toilet.

How and why do your priorities change?

Obviously, Mr Saddiq immediately becomes your priority. You need to ascertain if he has sustained an injury, assess why he has collapsed, make him safe and comfortable, and reassess your priorities of care in the light of your findings. Depending on the situation, this may cause you to reassess your priorities and communicate your revised plans to the people you are working alongside.

Exercise 7.11   Mental health

You are working on an acute psychiatric ward during the final management module of your course. It is decided that as part of your experience you will be in charge of the ward for the shift and be shadowed by the ward manager. The staff on duty includes a junior student nurse on their first ward placement, an experienced staff nurse who has worked on the ward for one year, and a new appointee health care assistant who started on the ward one week ago and is still trying to find her way around.

It is a 28-bedded unit divided into four bays. Today is Saturday and the ward is reasonably quiet as most patients are on weekend leave. The patients who are on the ward are mostly independent and self-caring. However, some patients are considered to be at risk.

Patient description	Planned and delegated care
James is 30 years old, married with two children. He has a recurrent history of bipolar disorder starting from when he was 19. His recent admission came about while he was decorating his home in the early hours of the morning while attempting to burn the waste wallpaper in the centre of the living room. His wife came downstairs to find the ground	
floor ablaze. The family only just escaped. He has been on the ward three days. He has a highly elevated mood, is excitable, and rapidly becomes frustrated with people who do not share his opinions. He has an inflated opinion of his own abilities that lead him to undertake dangerous undertakings. He has a rapidity of speech and quickly moves from one topic of conversation to the next. He has not slept in three days and states that he is too busy to sleep and does not need to eat, as he is invulnerable. He is hyperactive and sexually disinhibited.	
Helen is a 20-year-old young woman with a history of failed relationships and deliberate self-harming behaviour. She has numerous scars to the arms brought about by repeated self-mutilation. She has been on the ward for one month. While on the ward she has been sexually provocative with both staff and patients and consistently uses her physical appearance to draw attention to herself. She shows self-dramatization, theatricality, and exaggerated expression of emotion. Helen has a history of simulated convulsions to gain attention. She often considers her relationships more intimate than they actually are.	

Paul is a 45-year-old man who attempted to take his own life after the break-up of his marriage. He was admitted 10 days ago after taking an overdose of antidepressants. He has difficulty sleeping and often stays awake until the early hours of the morning. He is actively engaged in the ward activities and states that he now feels fine and does not know why he even attempted to take his own life. He is co-operative in his care, and warm and affable with the staff. He has decided to sort out his will and has asked to meet with his solicitor.

It is now evening visiting. The ward is beginning to fill with visitors and many of them wish to discuss their relative's care with the ward manager. The manager is in the ward office with a relative who is unhappy with the care that her father is receiving.

As you look down the ward, Helen, one of your patients, falls to the floor in front of a patient's relatives and begins to convulse. The relatives are very anxious and distressed and demand that you 'Do something to help her!' Helen's face is red and flushed.

As you attempt to deal with Helen's convulsion, James, another patient, becomes progressively more interfering. He attempts to take charge of the situation with Helen, becoming more and more agitated. His behaviour rapidly escalates and he becomes increasingly more aggressive to the surrounding relatives.

While you are trying to deal with the situation with Helen and James, the junior student nurse tells you that Paul has left the ward and she cannot find him anywhere.

 What would be your priorities in dealing with the above situation?

 How would you allocate your resources; that is, how would you use delegation?

 Consider the decisions that you would need to make in terms of delegation. What would be your reasons for those decisions?

Factors that can enhance or constrain decision making

The decisions that we make when nursing, or managing nursing, are often influenced by factors outside of our own personal control.

These can include:

- leadership/management styles

- hierarchical structures
- resources available
- knowledge deficits
- organizational systems
- policies and procedures
- statutory requirements
- risks you are willing to take.

Leadership/management styles

The three common leadership styles described by White and Lippitt (1960) cited in Marquis and Huston (2009) are described as authoritarian, *laissez-faire* and democratic leadership styles.

The authoritarian style of leadership reflects control, with communication flowing downwards from the leader, and decision making being instigated by the leader. This style of leadership does not encourage participation in decision making from staff and can stunt the growth of staff in terms of decision making and professional development.

The *laissez-faire* style of leadership is a permissive style, with little control, and distributes the responsibility for decision making among the team. As this style of leadership provides little or no direction, it can be very frustrating for a student who requires some support, direction and tuition with regard to decision making.

The democratic style of leadership focuses on involving others in decision making, emphasizing a team approach rather than an individualistic one. Support and guidance are key elements in this style of leadership, thus promoting growth within individuals. As a student, this style of leadership fits well with the concept of mentorship in nursing. Being aware of the predominant style of leadership in a placement can help you to identify what might be expected from you as a student, and can help you to understand the dynamics within the nursing team. This can help you to identify realistic expectations for yourself within the placement.

Hierarchical structures

Within hierarchical structures, the lower down the hierarchy that you are deemed to be, the less you will be encouraged to contribute to decision making. It is more likely that as a student you will be instructed in what to do, rather than encouraged to discuss the potential options available. Your approach to contributing to decision making might have to be adapted where the focus is on hierarchical structures. It may help to use reflection within your portfolio to identify how your decisions may have concurred with or differed from the person who made decisions about patient care, or how working within a hierarchy enhances or stunts motivation. It will also help to discuss your portfolio reflections with your mentor, peers and personal tutor.

Resources available

If you have access to all the resources you need when delivering care, the decisions you make can be made a little easier. However, if resources are scarce, this can lead to more complex decision making. For example, if the medical staff want to admit a patient from the emergency department who is medically unstable but you have no available bed on the ward, this may require you to make difficult decisions about which patient you will need to transfer to another area.

Knowledge deficits

If you have built up during your programme of study a sound knowledge base through attending classroom sessions, reading widely, actively learning from the staff you work with, reflecting on experiences, and developing action plans to increase your understanding of how to apply knowledge in practice, you will have developed a good foundation on which to base your decisions. If, however, you only do the minimum amount that will enable you to pass your practice outcomes/proficiencies and academic assignments, you will have less knowledge to draw on when faced with new situations that require you to make decisions, and may be more likely to make less effective decisions for your client group.

Organizational systems and policies and procedures

You need to get to know the organizational systems within which you work. Many organizations provide you with policies, procedures and guidelines that can be a useful aid with regard to decision making. There are also experts within organizations who provide both written guidance and the opportunity to seek advice from a specialist with regard to specific situations you encounter.

Most areas in which you work will have very useful policies and procedures that are written by experts that can be a valuable aid to both increase your knowledge and provide additional guidance that can aid your decision making. You will be required to use this knowledge and guidance within a specific situation, but they will help to increase your awareness of specific issues that you may not be familiar with on a day-to-day basis. This specialist knowledge will help to inform your decision making.

Statutory requirements

As a student nurse, you are required to have all evidence of medicine administration on a patient's prescription chart countersigned by a registered nurse. If your mentor says it does not matter, she is happy for you to sign the prescription chart and you decide to proceed, then you are both operating outside of statutory requirements. You have no evidence that you have not undertaken this task by yourself, and the mentor would be accountable for apparently letting you undertake a medicine round by yourself. Undertaking a medicine round and making decisions during the medicine round with your mentor at your side to sanction the decisions that you make can be an important learning experience.

Risks you are willing to take

This is a very difficult area. You may be tempted to leave the documenting of care until the end of your span of duty when you have undertaken all the care your patients require. However, if you decide to do this you may forget to document some aspects of care. This can mean that the care you have delivered remains omitted from the patients' records. The requirements are that your records are contemporaneous, therefore, your decision should always be to document care immediately after undertaking it.

You may be willing to take risks. However, whatever risks you take with regard to patient care, you must be prepared to be accountable for the decisions that you make.

Conclusion

In this chapter we have explored the transition to being a senior student nurse and what this means in terms of managing a group of patients rather than making decisions about individual care.

Managing care is an extremely complex skill. It requires you to think quickly, utilize resources effectively, be knowledgeable about your profession, work with others effectively and to be flexible and adaptable.

You also cannot divorce the decisions that you make in terms of management from the wider organization and this is something that is explored further in Chapter 8 in terms of making the transition to an accountable practitioner. You need to be aware of how you fit into the organization, and the parameters you need to work within.

References

Boucher, M. (1998) Delegation alert! *American Journal of Nursing*, 98(2): 26–32.

Bowers, B.J., Lauring, C. and Jacobson, N. (2001) How nurses manage time and work in long-term care, *Journal of Advanced Nursing*, 33(4): 484–91.

Hansten, R. and Washburn, M. (1996) Why don't nurses delegate? *Journal of Nursing Administration*, 26(12): 24–8.

Kalisch, B.J., Landstrom, G. and Williams, R.A. (2009) Missed nursing care: errors of omission, *Nursing Outlook*, 57(1): 3–9.

Marquis, B.L. and Huston, C.J. (2009) *Leadership Roles and Management Functions in Nursing*, 6th edn. London: Wolters Kluwer Health/Lippincott, Williams & Wilkins.

Nursing and Midwifery Council (NMC) (2008) *Advice on Delegation for Registered Nurses and Midwives.* London: NMC.

Price, B. (2008) Strategies to help nurses cope with change in the healthcare setting, *Nursing Standard*, 22(48): 50–6.

Royal College of Nursing (RCN) (2006) Supervision, accountability and delegation of activities to support workers: a guide for registered practitioners and support workers. Intercollegiate information paper developed by the CSP, RCSLT, BDA and the RCN, London.

Simon, E. (1998) Delegation competencies, *Nurse Educator*, 23(6): 47.

Siviter, B. (2008) *The Newly Qualified Nurse's Handbook*, Chapter 3. Philadelphia, PA: Elsevier.

Volker, D.L. (2003) Is there a unique nursing ethic? *Nursing Science Quarterly*, 16(3): 207–11.

Waterworth, S., May, C. and Luker, K. (1999) Clinical 'effectiveness' and 'interrupted' work, *Clinical Effectiveness in Nursing*, 3(4): 163–9.

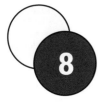

8 From student to staff nurse

- **Introduction**
- **Critical situations and intuition**
- **Helping others to learn**
- **Preventing complaints**
- **Why do complaints arise?**
- **Decision making and the transition to the status of a registered nurse**
- **Sign-off mentors for management students**
- **Preceptorship**
- **Expanded roles of the health care practitioner**
- **The path of lifelong learning**
- **Conclusion**
- **References**

Introduction

As you have worked through this book, you will have realized that decision making as a nurse is a very complex process; the pressure on nurses to make effective clinical decisions is enormous. You will by now, as a senior student nurse, appreciate that the burden of accountability is placed on you; that your decisions may well be challenged/investigated at any point and that you need to select up-to-date and appropriate evidence to support your practice.

Chapter 7 has highlighted the increasing complexity of decision making. The purpose of this chapter is to help you to make the transition from student to qualified nurse as this can prove to be an anxious time. Irrespective of the type of pre-registration course that students have followed, anxieties and misgivings about the type of preparation experienced have been reported by Maben and Macleod Clark, (1998); Charnley (1999); Gerrish (2000); Oermann and Garvin (2002); and O'Shea and Kelly (2007).

In this chapter the following elements are included to cover the period of transition from student to staff nurse:

- intuition
- helping others to learn
- helping to prevent complaints

- preceptorship
- lifelong learning skills.

You will also appreciate that as you move from student to qualified nurse that you will become fully accountable for your decisions, including those that concern delegation of work to others (as identified in Chapter 7). During your final placement as a student, you will still have your mentor near at hand to advise you; however, mentors will realize that you must now become independent in your decision making and will progressively take a 'back seat' to allow you to appreciate the intricacies of decision making at the level of a qualified nurse. Examine the example in Exercise 8.1 and think how you might deal with it; first as a student, then as a qualified nurse.

Exercise 8.1

A member of the medical staff persistently writes medication prescriptions unclearly.

 What actions could you take as a student?

 What actions could you take as a staff nurse/midwife?

The student, obviously still under supervision, will refer this to his or her mentor and perhaps will also ask the member of the medical staff to rewrite it in order that it can be read and administered safely.

A staff nurse, while carrying out the above course of action, will think long term and may well decide to take the matter further (with the involvement of a senior nurse manager) if the problem continues on the grounds that:

- this is an unacceptable risk to the patient
- medication policies clearly state that prescriptions must be legible
- this is a poor use of nursing time having to pursue an issue such as this.

This kind of event is an example of the (qualified) nurse's accountability to ensure safe and effective care for his or her patient. Think of what may occur if the matter is not resolved satisfactorily (there is evidence of a number of issues surrounding medication errors and their consequences) (Jones, 2009).

During investigations of events leading to medication errors, it has often been the case that while medical prescribers are held accountable, there has been a degree of accountability on the part of the nurse. This is the reason why the decision has to be to get the matter rectified in the short as well as the long term.

Critical situations and intuition

As you progress through your final placements, you will be exposed to more critical situations than previously. Your decision making will be to a large extent based on past experience in addition to the elements already incorporated from the 'add on framework'. You will, in the final stages of your pre-registration course, begin to acquire the elements of 'intuition'. This is a feature of an expert decision-maker. To illustrate this, consider the scenario in Exercise 8.2.

Exercise 8.2

You are working in a general surgical ward and are caring for a patient who had an exploratory laparotomy 24 hours ago after sustaining some abdominal injuries after a road traffic accident. A health care assistant has just taken his blood pressure and has found this to be very low. You go to see the patient who appears to be alert and talking to everyone.

You decide to monitor this patient very carefully – why?

You might well have encountered a similar situation in a previous clinical allocation. Having learned from this and perhaps reflected on it, you will have consolidated both your knowledge and experience. In this particular scenario, your underlying thought may be that the patient is at risk of developing a state of shock. (The low blood pressure is a clue.) You will obviously inform your mentor and probably the medical staff also. On the other hand, it could be the result of the administration of analgesia especially if it was an opioid. You will yourself perform a full set of vital signs: temperature, pulse respiration and blood pressure. You will repeat these at short intervals until the patient becomes more stable.

It is highly likely that intuition has played a role in this decision. As you acquire more experience, you will be using your intuition more and more. Intuition itself is a controversial topic within nursing. It has been the subject of a number of studies, particularly qualitative and has also been debated in the nursing literature. Much of the literature associates intuition with expert nursing practice (Benner and Tanner, 1987) but King and Appleton (1997: 200) in reviewing the literature surrounding the topic found that: 'Research would indicate that intuition appears to be used by members of every level of nursing from student to expert practitioner', and that, 'It has been established through ... studies that intuition is an integral part of the decision making process.'

Helping others to learn

The NMC (2008) expect that qualified nurses will assist co-workers to learn and expand their knowledge and skills. You also have a responsibility to ensure that individuals are competent to undertake the tasks you ask them to carry out. In addition, you need to ensure that individuals are following current policies and procedures as these often change in the light of new evidence and revisions to practice.

Exercise 8.3

You are working in a medical ward and working with you is a junior student nurse who is undertaking her first clinical placement. You would like her to carry out urinalysis as you have a number of patients recently admitted who require this as part of the admission and assessment process.

Having asked her politely if she knows how to do this, she maintains that she has been doing this for years as a health care assistant and can 'get on with it'.

Do you allow her to go ahead with the delegated task?

The student should have had input from the educational establishment that should indicate to her the correct procedure to be followed, but how do you know this? You will still need to check that she can perform this correctly.

Exercise 8.4

Which elements need to be assessed to ensure that the student can undertake this skill safely and accurately?

In working this out, you will find that this is a useful checklist for a short teaching session which, as a qualified nurse, you will need to undertake in the future (see Table 8.1).

You have a responsibility to ensure that the student carries this procedure out safely and correctly. If not, poor and unsafe practice may well continue and could result in incorrect diagnosis and treatment for a patient. As the person delegating the task, you will be held accountable for the decisions that you make and this includes the delegation of tasks to others.

In considering the elements you need to check for in relation to urinalysis, it could be useful to decide to convert this into a teaching and assessment tool that could be used by others.

Elements	Achieved	
	Yes	No
Follows prevention of infection precautions		
Ensures urine sample is fresh and uncontaminated		
Ensures reagent strips are in date and have been stored correctly		
Uses reagent strips correctly		
Interprets results correctly		
Safely disposes of urine and equipment		
Documents findings correctly		
Reports findings correctly		
Result *Achieved/Not achieved* (please delete as applicable)	**Signature**	**Date**

Table 8.1   Criteria for assessing urinalysis competence

In deciding to develop such a tool for the assessment of skills carried out routinely, you can help to ensure parity in teaching content and consistency with regard to assessments undertaken between yourself and other qualified staff. In using such a tool, the performance measured will yield consistent results. This means that the teaching and assessment will be both valid and reliable.

You can also advise the student to keep this assessment as portfolio evidence to support their achievement in practice.

Preventing complaints

There is no doubt that we now live in an increasingly litigious society. There are people and organizations that now make it their business to seek redress for deficiencies/errors in health care. Nurses often find themselves in the front line when faced with a complaining public.

While complaints are best prevented in the first place, the National Health Service (NHS) complaints procedure gives guidance on how to handle complaints that do arise. There is a need to address:

- time scales for responding to complaints
- the need for co-operation between social care and health care when complaints cross organizations who deliver care
- investigations and responses should be complainant-centred
- organizations need to produce annual reports regarding complaints received
- staff should know what to do if the complainant is dissatisfied.

Source: Hill Dickinson (2009).

Complaints need to be acknowledged within three working days, and a response to the complaint should be made within six months. This deadline may be extended but only with the agreement of the complainant. In addition, the person complaining, should be involved with the organization in how to proceed with the investigation.

Often, individuals receive care from both the NHS and Social Care. Where this is the case and the complaint involves both parties, one body should take the lead so that the complainant only has to deal with one organization. However, there should be co-operation between both organizations.

Annual reports of complaints and the issues raised should assist the organization to explore trends in complaints that should help the organization to address these. Complaints are an essential part of an organization's feedback mechanism, and can be an important educational tool for individuals as well as the organization (Norman, 2009).

If the person who has brought the complaint remains dissatisfied with the outcome of an investigation, the complainant still has the right to refer a case to the Health Service Ombudsman.

Consider the scenario in Exercise 8.5 with respect to how you might deal with a complaint.

Exercise 8.5

You are working in a clinical area where a number of elderly and confused clients are being cared for. One day the departmental manager receives a written complaint that had been sent to the trust complaints manager. The letter read as follows:

I am writing to complain about the care that my mother recently received on Ward X in your hospital. She was transferred from a nursing home with a small bedsore which the nursing home was working really hard to treat to heal this. When I visited her I found her to be confused, unkempt and her mouth was filthy as if she hadn't had a drink. I noticed her wedding ring and engagement ring were missing and I couldn't find these in her locker. Her supper tray was lying out of reach, untouched and cold. Her sheets had slipped off and her back and bottom were exposed as she was in a hospital gown. Whilst covering her up, I noticed that her bedsore had an offensive smell. I went to the desk to complain but the nurses were huddled together and obviously more interested in a magazine. When I eventually caught the attention of a nurse, I was told that my mother was not her patient. No effort was made to find my mother's nurse for me. When I said I could not wait any longer, the nurse I was talking to raised her eyebrows as if I was a nuisance.

I am really distressed about this, as my mother has always taken great pride in her appearance being a proud and independent lady.

(?) What decisions could have been made by the nursing staff that may have helped to avoid a complaint?

(?) What is the process that will be followed here?

(?) What lessons might be learned from this incident and how may such complaints be avoided in the future?

An investigation of this complaint will take place.

Why do complaints arise?

Complaints often arise from poor communication, poor handling of the situation and poor documentation contributes to such situations, but can lead to valuable insights into care (Norman, 2009). If you had to investigate this situation, what decisions would you make to act on this situation?

Resolution of complaints at the point of occurrence is perhaps the best way to try and deal with the matter. If successful, it can save a long and protracted investigation that is a costly item. An apology needs to be given, together with the reassurance that you will find out what has happened, and why. This may well help to diffuse this lady's anger and will reassure her that someone is listening to her and will follow the matter up.

It is also important to highlight different aspects that need investigating and possibly addressing in the letter of complaint. The aspects relate to:

- potential deficits in the nursing care delivered
- care of an individual's property
- lack of apparent interest and attention by the staff on duty.

It is important that you examine all documentation and talk to staff in order to ascertain why these things might have occurred and to take take action to resolve the issues even if you were not directly involved. This lady needs to be made aware of the time frame by which she should receive a response to her complaint. It is often the case that the complaint is not being made against you as an individual. Many nurses become very defensive when such an event occurs. This only serves to exacerbate the situation. However, it is important that complaints are acted on and improvements made to ensure such an event does not reoccur. It is also vital that feedback is given to the complainant, and that the feedback addresses all the issues highlighted in the letter of complaint.

The most effective way, however, is to ensure that adequate care is delivered to patients and that staff are aware of customer care approaches to people in order to prevent a complaint occurring in the first place. Ward managers should always examine their systems and observe their staff in action to explore if this could have been foreseen and hence prevented.

A written complaint such as this can also have implications for the wider organization as well as for yourself and so it is important that you think through the consequences of your actions and the decisions that you make.

Decision making and the transition to the status of a registered nurse

Your final clinical placement should help to build your overall confidence with respect to decision making. If you have worked through the relevant case studies (as applicable to your field of nursing/midwifery), reflected on these, incorporating stage by stage the 'add on framework' of decision making, you should be in a position as a qualified nurse to make your own independent decisions. As you make the transition to a registered nurse, you may, understandably, feel somewhat unsure about this. The accountability for your decisions now passes to you. Only you can answer for your decisions. This is probably what makes a number of nurses dread the day when they appear in the selected employment area as a qualified nurse/midwife. However, there will always be a more senior person to contact should you have any doubts about a difficult situation. Most areas do have a period of orientation into a job and it will be at this stage when you will have an opportunity to clarify issues with respect to decision making.

Sign-off mentors for management students

Your mentor in a management placement is a key person who will help you develop management skills and help to start that transition to a new registrant. They will also be a key player in helping you to develop your decision making abilities.

A sign-off mentor is an experienced mentor and practitioner who has the skills, knowledge and expertise to develop and assess your managerial abilities. The skills that the sign-off mentor has will be necessary to help you to develop your decision making abilities. The NMC (2008) also require a sign-off mentor to achieve additional criteria to those required of a mentor. These include being experienced in mentorship and having an in-depth understanding of accountability in relation to the decisions made in passing a student in practice at the end of the course. Sign-off mentors are usually the same individuals within a placement who fulfil the preceptorship role (see next section) and so they will be very aware of your development needs as a management student.

Exercise 8.6

Prior to your management placement, review your strengths and weaknesses with regard to decision making. It may be helpful to review your portfolio evidence and the comments that your mentor has made on your performance in previous placements.

Using your list, develop an action plan prior to your placement so that you can be proactive about your learning needs at your preliminary interview with the mentor.

This activity will assist you in articulating your learning needs to your sign-off mentor who can then facilitate opportunities whereby you can develop your decision making abilities.

You need to constantly seek out informal as well as formal feedback as to how your abilities are developing. Remember, you will be operating at the third stage of the 'add on framework' of decision making. At this stage you need to be initiating and taking more responsibility for the decisions that you are making. This does not mean that you do not consult with your mentor. It does mean you need to think about the decisions that you will make, and ask the sign-off mentor to verify your course of action. The mentor is still accountable for you at this stage.

Preceptorship

The NMC (2006) recommends that all new registrants have a period of preceptorship to help practise in accordance with the Code (NMC, 2008) and to develop confidence and competence in the registrant role. Some trusts have had preceptorship schemes in operation for some time. However, it is now recommended that all employers of new registrants have a preceptorship scheme in place.

Preceptorship is a way of using role modelling to support learning and growth of individuals (Canadian Nursing Association, 2004). From the definition you can see that preceptorship is similar in many ways to mentorship, but the term 'preceptorship' within the UK is utilized for support for the new registrant.

In order to facilitate role modelling to support learning, the preceptor needs to be someone who is:

- confident in their practice
- sensitive to the needs of patients/clients
- an effective team member
- up to date with knowledge and practice.

Source: NMC (2006).

The NMC (2006) also go on to say that preceptors need to provide honest, objective and positive feedback to the new registrant in order to help to build on their knowledge and skills, as well as to enhance the new registrant's confidence.

Exercise 8.7

What do you think the differences are between having a mentor and a preceptor?

The roles of guide and facilitator of learning are very similar. However, the preceptor does not have a formal, summative role in terms of assessing their preceptee in the way that a mentor has to judge a student's performance in practice. The main difference though is that the mentor is accountable for the student's actions whereas accountability for actions will always lie with the registrant who undertook those actions, or made specific decisions regarding care.

It is generally felt that preceptorship schemes can ease the transition from student to qualified nurse. A study by Amos (2001: 41) carried out to evaluate the role transition from student to staff nurse identified the fact that: 'structured supervision by preceptors and rotation programmes were the most beneficial ways to assist role transition'.

With respect to decision making, such a scheme can help to build the confidence and competencey of the newly registered nurse. The first six months as a registrant can be particularly stressful (Charnley, 1999) with Kramer (2004) identifying this period as 'reality shock'. Makepeace (1999) highlighted that the biggest change from being a student to a staff nurse/midwife is the sense of responsibility. This is particularly relevant to decision making. Preceptorship cannot completely eliminate reality shock and stress, but it can help to minimize it for an individual if the preceptor is supportive and approachable. There is a real need to minimize stress as it can be a significant factor in new registrants leaving the profession (Bick, 2000).

Special support in the form of preceptorship when making the transition to new registrant status is crucial in successful adjustment, and can help to pave the way towards positive and stable career experiences (Nash et al., 2009).

With preceptorship, there is an opportunity for the gradual development of skills, confidence and competence in relation to the decisions that you make. Having someone you can trust, whom you can use as a sounding board for your decisions, and who will give constructive advice and feedback is absolutely invaluable.

Exercise 8.8

As a preceptee, what do you think your responsibilities are within the preceptorship relationship?

Your list of responsibilities may be quite personal to you but you should certainly have included:

- the need to identify specific learning needs and an action plan to address these needs
- your need to be aware of what your employer expects of you by reviewing your job description
- your need to reflect on your practice experience and seek feedback from your preceptor on your performance
- your need to continue to keep a portfolio of learning.

Source: Adapted from NMC (2006).

Exercise 8.9

What do you think will be the main stresses and challenges for you as a new registrant in terms of decision making?

The stresses and challenges will probably be personal to you as an individual. You need to use your preceptor wisely by disclosing to them your fears such as your perceived lack of knowledge or expertise, lack of specific experience and limits in your competence. You should also use them to increase your knowledge of what you are allowed to do by the organization in which you work. Oermann and Garvin (2002) highlight within their research that new registrants find that some of the greatest challenges relate to applying knowledge to practice situations, and the need to improve their clinical judgement. They also go on to say that a trusting and supportive relationship between the preceptor and yourself makes the learning less stressful. Hence, your preceptor can be the key to continued, successful development.

Expanded roles of the health care practitioner

Another element that often causes concern to the newly qualified nurse/midwife is the undertaking of an expansion to the practice role (i.e. intravenous medications). Historically, this may have been an aspect of care that nurses became responsible for some time after qualification. However, with the reduction in junior doctors' hours, it is often the case that this aspect of care is taken on fairly soon after qualification in acute hospital trusts. Most trusts have learning packages to enable the newly qualified nurse to take on this role and competence in practice has to be established. However, this aspect of care can prove problematic if the newly qualified nurse is not alert to some of the difficulties surrounding this issue. Consider the scenario in Exercise 8.10.

Exercise 8.10

A patient needs intravenous flucloxacillin. It has been administered before but you have noticed on a previous occasion that this particular patient has developed a respiratory wheeze shortly after administration. Something tells you (intuition again!) that all is not well.

Do you go ahead and give the dose?

You may be thinking that the patient has become sensitized to this medication. You are also aware that the intravenous route can cause a rapid allergic reaction. You do not feels happy about this. Even as a qualified nurse you still have the right to non-involvement in the task if you feel that there is a problem that is outside your competence. How might you proceed in this situation?

You could contact the medical staff to let them know of the problem and leave it to them to decide how to proceed – they might decide to alter the medication or give it themselves; they may diagnose the wheeze as a different cause other than the medication but only they can make such a decision. If they instruct you to go ahead, you could ask for them to be present when the medication is given as they could help to deal with any problem that results. As a follow-up, it might be worth having a discussion with a pharmacist to see what their advice might be in similar situations.

The above scenario does illustrate the altered accountability for a qualified nurse. The important issue is to get advice regarding your decision in such a case. If you are unhappy, do not yield to pressure; sometimes nurses are made to feel that they are causing an unnecessary fuss – provided you state your case (with knowledge) and in a polite way, then your decision cannot reasonably be challenged. This is the sort of situation that you may wish to discuss with your preceptor.

The path of lifelong learning

As a senior student and a new registrant, you may feel that you should know everything there is to know. However, if you discuss this with other registrants and ask them about their experiences, they will be able to reassure you that this is not the case. In fact, nurses and midwives who are very experienced will still tell you that they are still learning. They will also be able to share their experiences of feeling they should be fully competent, while feeling that they know very little.

However, in order to make safe and sensible decisions as a qualified nurse, you do need to keep yourself up to date. In fact, the NMC requires this of you in order to keep your registration 'live' and they may ask for evidence of this when you need to re-register on an annual basis. Lifelong learning as a qualified nurse is a requirement. The nature of your further learning will depend on your employment and what you must ensure is that you keep a current portfolio of evidence. As a student nurse you were required to keep such a document, elements of which you shared with your tutors and mentors.

The decisions that you make as a qualified nurse provide a rich resource of reflection and learning while you are a qualified nurse. It is particularly important that as a profession we learn from our decisions, both positive or negative events. There is always a risk involved when caring for people and our task as qualified nurses and midwives is to minimize the risks. This is where policies, procedures and guidelines are produced by health care trusts to ensure that care is of the correct standard. We have emphasized in the 'add on framework' the necessity of incorporating such policies into our decision-making from a fairly early stage and, if you have done this, then as a qualified nurse, you will appreciate their importance. In addition, you need to continue to read current literature and research as developments in these areas continually affect the way in which we should practise.

Conclusion

Making the transition from being a student to a new registrant can be extremely stressful but you should now be able to appreciate that the transition can be made less stressful with the help of a preceptor, and through continuing to develop your knowledge and expertise.

Becoming a nurse/midwife is an exciting time in your career, but you need to remember that it is not the end of learning and it is certainly not the end of supportive relationships that can help you to develop. There are always other health care staff and managers with whom you can consult to ascertain that you have chosen the right course of action if you are unsure.

Becoming a new registrant is the first step you take in your qualified role, and the success of your career will depend on your willingness to learn from your experiences.

References

Amos, D. (2001) An evaluation of staff nurse role transition, *Nursing Standard*, 16(3): 36–41.

Benner, P. and Tanner, C. (1987) How expert nurses use intuition, *American Journal of Nursing*, 87(1): 23–31.

Bick, C. (2000) Please help! I'm newly qualified, *Nursing Standard*, 14(16): 33–6.

Canadian Nurses Association (2004) *Achieving Excellence in Professional Practice: A Guide to Preceptorship and Mentoring.* Ottawa: Canadian Nurses Association.

Charnley, E. (1999) Occupational stress in the newly qualified staff nurse, *Nursing Standard*, 13(29): 33–6.

Gerrish, C. (2000) Still fumbling along? A comparative study of the newly qualified nurse's perception of the transition from student to staff nurse, *Journal of Advanced Nursing*, 32(2): 473–80.

Hill Dickinson (2009) *The New NHS Complaints Procedure Explained – April 2009.* Available online at www.hilldickinson.com (accessed 27 November 2009).

Jones S.W. (2009) Reducing medication administration errors in nursing practice, *Nursing Standard*, 23(50): 40–6.

King, L. and Appleton, J.V. (1997) Intuition: a critical review of the research and rhetoric, *Journal of Advanced Nursing*, 26(1): 194–202.

Kramer, M. (2004) *Reality Shock: Why Nurses Leave Nursing.* St Louis, MO: Mosby.

Maben, J. and Macleod Clark, J. (1998) Project 2000 diplomates' perceptions of their experiences of transition from student to staff nurse, *Journal of Clinical Nursing*, 7(2): 145–53.

Makepeace, A. (1999) Reality bites, *Nursing Times*, 95(16): 60.

Nash, R., Lemcke, P. and Sacre, S. (2009) Enhancing transition: an enhanced model of clinical placement for final year nursing students, *Nurse Education Today*, 21(1): 48–56.

Norman, A. (2009) Involving nurses in the complaints process leads to more effective care, *Nursing Times*, 105(44): 11.

Nursing and Midwifery Council (NMC) (2006) *Preceptorship Guidelines,* Circular 21/2006. London: NMC.

Nursing and Midwifery Council (NMC) (2008) *Advice on Delegation for Registered Nurses and Midwives.* London: NMC.

Oermann, M.H. and Garvin, M.F. (2002) Stresses and challenges for new graduates in hospitals, *Nurse Education Today*, 22(3): 225–30.

O'Shea, M. and Kelly, B. (2007) The lived experiences of newly qualified nurses on clinical placement during the first six months following registration in the Republic of Ireland, *Journal of Clinical Nursing*, 16(8): 1534–42.

Index

The index entries appear in word-by-word alphabetical order.

A BEGINNER'S GUIDE TO EVIDENCE-BASED PRACTICE IN HEALTH AND SOCIAL CARE

Helen Aveyard; Pam Sharp

"I would just like to say this is the best text I have come across for my module for under-graduate students. It is pitched at just the right level and is written in a style that is easy to engage with. The layout and the structure are also easy to follow and it is a really good introduction to EBP. I intend recommending this to my students and thank you once again for sending me a copy of this."

Jean Davison, Teesside University, UK

Have you heard of 'evidence based practice' but don't know what it means?

Are you having trouble relating evidence to your practice?

This is the book for anyone who has ever wondered what evidence based practice is or how to relate it to practice. This accessible book presents the topic in a simple, easy to understand way, enabling those unfamiliar with evidence based practice to apply the concept to their practice and learning.

Using everyday language, this book provides a step by step guide to what we mean by evidence based practice and how to apply it. It also:

- Provides an easy to follow guide to searching for evidence
- Explains how to work out if the evidence is relevant or not
- Explores how evidence can be applied in the practice setting
- Outlines how evidence can be incorporated into your academic writing

A Beginner's Guide to Evidence Based Practice in Health and Social Care is key reading for everyone involved in looking at and applying evidence – students, practice educators, mentors and practising health and social care professionals.

Contents: *Acknowledgements – Introduction – What is evidence based practice? – The development of evidence based practice When do we need to use evidence and what evidence do we need? – What are the different types of research? – How do I find the evidence to support my practice and learning? – How do I know if the evidence is convincing and useful? – How to use and implement evidence in your practice and learning – References – Appendix A – Glossary – Appendix B Useful Web Links*

2009 224pp
978-0-335- 23603–9 (Paperback) 978-0-335- 23602–2 (Hardback)

A PRACTICAL GUIDE TO CARE PLANNING IN HEALTH AND SOCIAL CARE

Marjorie Lloyd

'A valuable resource which will capture the interest of all those involved in planning high quality care.'
C.Dickie, Lecturer of Adult Nursing, University of the West of Scotland, UK

This accessible guide takes the mystery and fear out of care planning and will help you to develop a person centred approach to delivering good quality nursing care in all clinical settings. The book explores each part of the care planning process in detail and provides opportunities for you to reflect upon practice and to develop effective skills through:

- Interprofessional working
- Risk management
- Communication and listening skills
- Reflection
- Supervision

Practical examples demonstrate how best to complete care planning documents and samples are provided in the appendix for you to practice with. Useful websites and checklists are included to help you become more confident with the care planning process. *A Practical Guide to Care Planning in Health and Social Care* is essential reading for all health and social care students involved in planning good quality care. A structured plan is the essential foundation for the delivery of safe and effective care.

This publication successfully guides the reader through the stages of care planning using a simple yet systematic approach. Its strength lies in the carefully designed format which gives consideration to the evidence base as well as providing guidance for the practical application of care plans.

Contents: *Introduction to the Care Planning Process – The Assessment of Needs – Planning care with the individual in need – Glossary – Recommended Reading – Websites for further information and advice – References – Appendix – Index*

March 2010 160pp
978-0-335- 23732–6 (Paperback) 978-0-335- 23731–9 (Hardback)

REFLECTIVE PRACTICE FOR HEALTHCARE PROFESSIONALS 3/e

Beverley J. Taylor

"Reflection, as a process of critical self-evaluation, continues to grow and be recognised as a successful, approach to improving, changing and managing healthcare practice. This latest text by Taylor is a welcome addition to the increasing body of knowledge on the subject. She writes, as always, with exceptional clarity and manages to combine practical guidance with experiential insights and theoretical frameworks. Highlighting the importance of ordinary human communication for all healthcare professionals, Taylor's text and presence is anything but ordinary.'

Professor Dawn Freshwater, University of Leeds, UK

This popular book provides practical guidance for healthcare professionals wishing to reflect on their work and improve the way they undertake clinical procedures, interact with other people at work and deal with power issues.

The new edition has been broadened in focus from nurses and midwives exclusively, to include all healthcare professionals.

Practice stories by a variety of healthcare professionals are interweaved throughout the book to illustrate reflective practice and 'author's reflections' boxes are used to illustrate the author's experience of reflective practice.

The book contains a clear and comprehensive description of:

- The fundamentals of reflective practice and how and why it is embraced in healthcare professions
- Strategies for effective reflection
- Systematic approaches to technical, practical and emancipatory reflection
- A step-by-step guide to applying the Taylor REFLECT model

This edition also introduces the concept of 'ordinariness' in health care, which used consciously with the reflective practice processes in this book should increase the likelihood that patients receiving healthcare will feel acknowledged, heard and comforted as intelligent human beings.

Contents: *Introduction – The nature of reflection and practice – Preparing for reflection and the REFLECT model – Types of reflection – Technical reflection – Practical reflection – Emancipatory reflection - Applying Taylor's REFLECT model to practice – Reflective practice in research and scholarship – Being human and reflection as a lifelong process – References – Index*

2010 240pp
978-0-335- 23835–4 (Paperback)

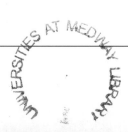